# CONTENTS

# INTRODUCTION

The intention for this book is to attempt to objectify the phenomenon referred to as "chronic pain" and provide a method to release it. Chronic Pain is an extremely interesting phenomenon, which all people experience to some extent.

As we go through life, we will certainly experience "painful moments", either physical (injury) or emotional. Until these moments are correctly "processed", they will exist in our body and mind as a source of "chronic pain". Physically, as chronic muscular tension. Emotionally, as "unconscious" fear, guilt, regret, rage and so on. Mentally, as confusion, racing thoughts, overwhelm and so on.

If never consciously processed, chronic pain will persist until death. That doesn't seem desirable. Regardless of how much chronic pain one is currently enduring, whether they are haunted, traumatized, or merely bothered, it seems rational to understand how to actively process and release pain, and thus be "free" of it. Life would certainly be better without lingering pain, would it not?

The active process by which a painful moment ceases to be painful is the process of "consciousness". By the active process of consciousness, we "become conscious" of the finite subset of reality that we have so far experienced.

The painful moments in our lives are the most difficult to become conscious of because each moment demands that we accept that reality is not that which we wish it to be. People we love have died or gone away, we have been physically hurt, we have been betrayed, our status has been diminished, we have been humiliated, our embarrassing weaknesses and faults have become known, and so on.

It is true -- our chances of surviving, of obtaining and achieving our dreams, of using our body to its potential, of experiencing joy, have all been diminished during the painful moments of our lives.

But the state we all know that we desire deep down - enlightenment, self-esteem, self-actualization, individuation, nirvana, the "clear state" (it goes by many names) - demands that we become conscious of all moments of our lives.

The process of "consciousness" is neither immediate, automatic nor trivial. It is an active process of perceiving, conceptualizing and objectifying. It involves actively feeling physical tensions in the body, allowing inhibited emotions to express, contemplating painful memories, and reorganizing one's convictions about objective reality to be in harmony with it.

As one releases more pain, by the process of consciousness, valuable states of being such as tranquility, joy, confidence, inspiration, and so on, become more common, and eventually the "default". There becomes time for such states, because no longer is every moment held captive by swirling, chronic fear, rage, guilt, regret and other unprocessed chronic pain.

The most common sources of pain are physical injuries, conflict with others, and metaphysical contemplation. The last is often overlooked. It is the "angst" of a person struggling to make sense of themselves, reality, and their relationship to reality.

With little understanding of the process of consciousness, low self-esteem and fear of pain itself, pain that would ideally be temporary, becomes chronic. That is to say that it is evaded, unchecked, denied, buried, repressed. This process of "evasion" operates simultaneously physically, emotionally and mentally, meaning that we simultaneously evade the physical sensations of pain, we evade the emotions of pain, and we evade the thoughts of pain.

To release chronic pain, we must replace the chronic habitual process of evasion, which maintains pain, with the process of consciousness.

This book presents 3 tools which are intended to help you release pain, and achieve self-esteem and a clear state of mind.

The first tool is simply knowledge of a model of reality pertaining to pain, consciousness, memory, muscular tension, emotion and thought.

The second tool is a set of exercises to help you notice chronic muscular tensions, and inefficient movement patterns. They come at the end of each chapter. You can do them whenever you want. You can skip them, do them out of order, repeat your favorites. Or you can just do them according to the order in which I've written them. It's all up to you, and probably makes no difference.

None of these exercises are "special". They were selected fairly arbitrarily from a pool of hundreds, if not thousands, of equally valuable exercises. I have included 9 exercises, which should be sufficient for someone to get the "idea" behind the exercises, so they can create their own.

The third tool is a method for initiating and maintaining the process of consciousness.

That method is, essentially, slow, calm movements with deep attentive focus on the muscles. These movements allow you to perceive and become conscious of chronic "tensions" in your musculature, which are directly associated with emotional pain and mental conflict.

The chronic muscular tensions in your body can be considered to be the "gateway" to the emotions and thoughts associated with painful moments in your life. These emotions and thoughts are not usually accessible. Even therapy generally "beats around the bush", with embarrassingly low success, while accessing the "soul" through the body is literally a "sure thing".

This method is not a 5 minute miracle. In fact, the first time you try it, you may get no results whatsoever, and you will be tempted to think "this doesn't work". However, if you stick with it, you will most likely learn to do it successfully.

At the end of each chapter you will be provided with movements that will train your ability to perceive and control your muscles. This will form the foundation for attempts to release pain, which becomes easier, the better your perception and control become.

The following problems could improve: muscular pain, joint stiffness, tendinopathy, cold extremities, shakiness, lack of focus, headaches, shallow breathing, misaligned spine, poor posture, low energy, overwhelm, feeling tired all the time, thyroid, low testosterone (men), anxiety, chronic guilt and regret, repressed rage, phobias, stress, neurosis, psychosis, and more.

The following values could develop: balance, flexibility, spontaneity, grace, strength, movement, courage, rationality, assertiveness, confidence, self-esteem, intelligence, productiveness, mental clarity, calmness, vigour, libido, blood flow, sexual sensitivity, presence, passion, intention, awareness, concentration, purpose, lightness, pride, happiness, and more.

It's easy to confidently make such claims in this case because our topic is releasing trapped pain from the body, which is certainly a real thing, and has been done successfully for millennia. It is practically intuitive that releasing trapped pain can immediately improve your life in many ways.

This book should not be taken as intended to be an accurate description of objective reality. While this book may appear to deal with the sciences of biology and neurology, it is more so a philosophical work, dealing with the sciences of metaphysics (the science of being), and epistemology (the science of acquiring and verifying knowledge).

Metaphysics and epistemology are both very immature sciences, and neither have progressed far enough to accurately explain observations. Therefore, this presents merely a model for your contemplation. Regardless of how accurate the model is, I'm sure that learning it will be worthwhile, and valuable to your life.

The source materials for this book are:

- Character Analysis, by Wilhelm Reich
- Bioenergetics, by Alexander Lowen
- Objectivism, by Ayn Rand
- Dianetics, by L. Ron Hubbard
- Beyond Systems, by Egwin Ertl
- Vahva Fitness, by Eero Westerberg
- Zen Buddhism, as described by Alan Watts

I would certainly like to thank these people for writing down such great thoughts, as they have been immensely valuable to my life. I would also like to thank my girlfriend, Alina, and my family, for their contributions, both to this book and my life.

# CHAPTER 1: MUSCULAR PAIN IS NOT WHAT WE'VE BEEN TAUGHT

We must begin with the physical component of pain. There are two reasons for this. The first reason is that the physical seems to be the easily accessible "gateway" to emotions and thoughts. The second reason is that it is the part of pain about which people have so many perniciously incorrect beliefs. Having false beliefs about muscular pain will make it impossible to ever release pain and a desirable way of living.

Chronic muscular pain is not what we've been taught to believe it is. We were taught, as soon as we began to investigate muscular pain, that it is a condition of the muscles themselves.

We were taught that muscular pain involves "tight", "inflamed" muscles. Possibly with "adhesions" and "scar tissue". And therefore, it made total sense when we were taught that the correct treatment is to stretch them, to take anti-inflammatories, to get massaged in order to soften the muscles and "break up the scar tissue".

We were taught about causes. That muscular pain is caused by such things as "repetitive strain injury", where the muscles are used too much, and "inactivity", where the muscles are used too little. We were taught that "bad posture" causes muscular pain, as does "moving incorrectly". Sitting wrong, standing wrong, bending wrong, squatting wrong, lying down wrong, holding your head wrong, holding your shoulders wrong.... and so on.

However, this is all mythology. It is entirely false information. False, because it looks only at the symptoms of muscular pain and doesn't even begin to address anything close to a root cause. This book is about tracking the root cause all the way down to its depths.

Every single day, probably more than a billion people ingest false information about muscular pain from people who call themselves "massage therapists", "physiotherapists", "personal trainers", "doctors", "sports physicians", "chiropractors", and so many other names. Recently, "Fitness YouTubers" are heavily involved.

What do their teachings all have in common? Every single one of these people believes that muscular pain is caused physically and should be treated physically. Because of this belief, literally almost every person in the world believes that their muscular pain has some physical cause, and they seek a physical solution.

Even in the case of a destructive physical injury, while of course the acute, transient muscular pain is caused physically, the chronic muscular pain that persists years or decades later, long after physical tissues have had a chance to heal, is no longer of physical cause.

If you were to go onto YouTube and search "neck pain", or "back pain" or "hip pain", or any other "pain" term related to muscles or joints, you will find an unlimited supply of videos about how muscular pain is caused by bad posture, inactivity, sitting too much, bending wrong, repetitive strain injury, and so on, and then repeating the same old tired false solutions.

The most common false solutions are stretching, foam rolling, lacrosse ball rolling, strengthening and "activating". If this stuff really worked, you would have already been cured a long time ago. The continued existence of your muscular pain is evidence that the solutions you've been exposed to thus far are incorrect.

The endemic fiction about muscular pain began around the 1950s. A physician by the name of Vladimir Janda, creator of the "Janda" approach, introduced an incorrect theory called "The Theory of Muscular Imbalance".

This theory states that pain occurs when some muscles in the body become tight and overactive, while others become weak and underactive. Therefore, the solution is to stretch the tight, overactive muscles, and strengthen the weak, underactive muscles.

This theory has held progress in the treatment of muscular pain back for decades. Why? Because it's quite easy to understand, easy to explain and seems to make so much sense.

Two major applications of the theory are "Upper Cross Syndrome" and "Lower Cross Syndrome".

In the supposed "Upper Cross Syndrome", the upper back is slouched and the neck is pulled forward due, supposedly due to tight chest muscles, and weak upper back muscles. Therefore, the prescribed solution is to stretch the chest muscles, and strengthen the upper back muscles.

In the supposed "Lower Cross Syndrome", the pelvis is tilted forward and the lower back is excessively curved, supposedly due to tight hip flexors and weak glutes. Therefore, the prescribed solution is to stretch the hip flexors, and strengthen the glutes.

See how much sense this makes? An innocent visitor to the physiotherapist assumes that the physiotherapist has a correct understanding of muscular pain, and so when the physiotherapist confidently explains this incorrect model, the patient thinks they're hearing the truth.

The patient thus goes to perform stretches and strengtheners as instructed, but it's almost certain that they'll be back, under the assumption that they didn't work hard enough, didn't stick to the routine, or didn't do the exercises correctly. The physiotherapist either explains again or suggests "maybe it's a different muscle that is the root cause, and that's the one we need to target!"

Often the patient ends up on an absurd quest to correctly identify the root-cause dysfunctional muscle in their body and may remain on this quest for decades. They search for the perfect stretch, or the perfect strengthener, which will make the pain go away.

Unfortunately, it will never be found. Why? Because there is no stretch or strengthener that will heal muscle pain. Because stretching and strengthening are purely physical approaches, and therefore cannot interface with the root cause of muscular pain.

Vladimir Janda did actually begin to move toward the truth late in his career, but very few people know about this. Janda at least suspected that the cause of muscular imbalances comes from the central nervous system. And he did come up with exercises that take this into account. Exercises that address balance, stability and coordination began to appear.

However, even though this an innovation in the correct direction, it was for the most part, totally ignored. And all that really survives is the "stretch and strengthen" model. Today, "professionals" rummage around the body finding weak muscles and tight muscles, prescribing strengtheners and stretches, while also "massaging" the muscles.

Be aware, that for someone with muscular pain, generally all muscles are weak, tight, shortened and chronically contracted. There are no muscles of the body that are in good order. Not a single one. For one muscle to be in good order, all muscles need to be in good order.

**Summary of this chapter:**

- Almost all fitness advisors take a "purely physical approach"
- The believe that muscular pain is a condition of the muscles themselves
- The Theory of Muscular Imbalance is the central theory of purely physical approaches
- Stretching and strengthening, as purely physical approaches, cannot heal muscular pain

**Exercise 1: Smile**

There is almost certainly significant chronic muscular tension in the muscles of your face. Your ability to do many, if not all, facial expressions is prevented by chronic muscular tensions that were voluntarily ordered during the many experiences of your life, limit expression, limit feeling and limit action.

As you learn to smile, you will learn the nature of the chronic muscular tensions that inhibit your potential for a natural, wonderful smile. As you become aware of such tensions, you will accept that tensions also limit all facial expressions, and all bodily expressions.

Begin with a small smile. Pull the corners of your mouth apart, while leaving your lips sealed. Focus deeply on the muscles around your face and try to notice any tension. Ask yourself, "what is that tension? Why do I feel it?"

After you have explored that experience, move to a huge smile. Smile fiercely with every muscle of your face. Again, notice tensions and ask yourself what the tension is and why it exists.

Eventually, you may look at yourself in the mirror while you do these smiling exercises. Observe your face and ask yourself, "Why does my face look like that? What does my facial expression reflect about my character and my way of living?" Remind yourself that everything is OK and realize that in the future your smile and face may come to resemble your ideal vision of them.

# CHAPTER 2: HOLDING MUSCLES IN A CONSTANT STATE OF TENSION

In the book "Relax Into Stretch", author Pavel Tsoutsaline makes a statement that has probably pushed some people in the correct direction. Please note that I do not recommend any other teachings by Tsoutsaline.

Tsoutsaline pointed out that muscles often refuse to lengthen not because of a physical condition of the muscles, but because the brain is holding them contracted (by means of the nervous system). Notice how this relates to Janda's later theory, that muscular pain comes from the central nervous system.

Tsoutsaline suggested that the brain holds muscles tight to prevent you moving into a position that the brain deems "unsafe". For example, consider the side splits. Imagine sliding your feet outward, with the muscles of your inner thigh and groin stretching out. You'll reach a point where you don't seem to be able to go any further.

He is suggesting that the brain is holding your inner thigh muscles and groin muscles tense here, because it detects that if you were to go any further, the lack of control and coordination could result in injury. So, he suggests "waiting out the tension", giving the brain time to understand that the position is "safe", and when it does so, it will turn off some of the contraction and allow the muscles to lengthen.

There is one thing that he gets correct. Fear can prevent you from moving in ways that could produce pain. However, he refers to an extremely specific case, that is really only applicable to a gymnast, dancer or martial artist. One who already is generally free of muscular pain, and simply wishes to require extreme flexibility.

If a regular person tries to apply Tsoutsaline's idea, they will make a tiny amount of progress, as some of their muscular pain is related to the issue that Tsoutsaline describes, however, this issue is probably 1/10000th of the overall picture. Someone with muscle pain is likely to gain more flexibility with Tsoutsaline's method, but unlikely to significantly decrease pain.

Tsoutsaline is correct that the brain can hold muscles contracted to prevent unwanted outcomes, however he suggests only one unwanted outcome. That outcome being "injury in extreme positions". The brain, having a fear of "injury in extreme positions", holds the muscles tight to keep the body from moving into those extreme positions.

However, the brain can hold the muscles tight for many reasons. In fact, whenever a muscle is chronically tight and painful, it's because the brain is chronically contracting that muscle.

But what does that mean, really? What does it mean to say, "the brain is contracting a muscle"? Is the brain some renegade organ with a will of its own, outside of our conscious control? Is chronic muscular contraction, and chronic muscular pain caused by a part of our brain over which we have no control?

To answer this, we should consult the anatomy and neurology of the body.

Any muscle in your body is made up of approximately hundreds of thousands of muscle fibers. These muscle fibers are divided up into groups, with each group containing a few hundred muscle fibers.

Each of these groups forms what is referred to by neurologists as a "motor unit", with its own "motor neuron", which is connected to the "motor cortex" in your brain.

So, the path from brain to muscle is (1) Motor Cortex, (2) Motor Neuron, (3) Neuromuscular Junction, (4) Muscle Fiber Group

Whenever you want to move, a signal is sent from the Motor Cortex, down the Motor Neurons to the required muscle fibers, causing them to contract. Aside from sudden reflex reactions, which have nothing to do with chronic muscular tension, this is the only way muscles can be made to contract.

When muscles are constantly tight and painful, it is because the motor cortex is sending constant, round the clock signals to the muscles to remain contracted.

Now for a shock. The Motor Cortex and the motor neurons form a part of the central nervous system called the "Somatic Nervous System". Somatic means "of or related to the body".

However, the Somatic Nervous System also goes by another name - The Voluntary Nervous System. It's called the voluntary nervous system because you have conscious voluntary control over it. It responds to your will.

The movement of your body, and the contraction of your muscles is under your conscious, voluntary control. If a muscle is contracted, it's because the owner of that muscle has chosen to keep it contracted.

If your lower back is tight and chronically contracted, it is because you have made the conscious choice to contract it.

If your neck and shoulders are tight, it's because you're squeezing them.

If your knees or hips are stiff, it's because you're locking them in place.

If the arches of your feet are sore, it's because you're squeezing them.

A few questions should be arising in your mind.

Why would you choose to contract a muscle in the first place? Why would you continue to hold it contracted? Why can't you simply "let it go"?

It is at this point that this book really becomes interesting. Up until this point, I've had to deal with dismantling decades of false dogma about muscular pain, simply to reach the root cause of chronic muscular pain -- your own conscious instructions to hold your muscles chronically contracted.

I'll make that statement extremely clear:

When your muscles are chronically tight and painful, it's because you have made a voluntary, conscious choice to hold your muscles in a state of constant tension.

**Summary of this chapter:**

- The brain sends impulses through your nervous system to your muscles to make them contract
- The brain can hold muscles tight to "protect" you
- If a muscle in your body is tight, it's because you're chronically squeezing it
- Chronic muscle squeezing is a voluntary conscious choice (made in the past)

## Exercise 2: Static Hold for Arms and Legs

Significant chronic muscular tension most likely exists in the muscles of your legs, pelvic area, lower back and shoulders. This tension makes it impossible to move gracefully, attractively, vigorously, purposefully and so on.

Stand with your feet under your hip joints (most likely approximately 8 inches) and the inside edges of your feet parallel. Bend your knees slightly so that your pelvis dips directly downward about 4 inches. Hold your arms out in front of you, with a comfortable bend in your elbows, and your palms facing your face.

Hold this position so that you begin to notice your muscles struggling. Notice which muscles begin to struggle. Resist the urge to give up at the first sensation of soreness or fatigue.

Ask yourself, "Am I using my muscles with optimum efficiency? Am I using optimum patterns of muscular contraction to support this movement? Or am I using old, inefficient patterns, which I could improve right now?"

Attempt to improve the way you hold yourself to be more efficient and comfortable. Let go of any "image" you have of how the position should look, and instead let your perception be your guide.

Hold until you feel like you need to stop. 20 minutes would be great, but 5 is also great, as is only 2 or 1. Put the criteria for success simply on watching your muscles and noticing feelings.

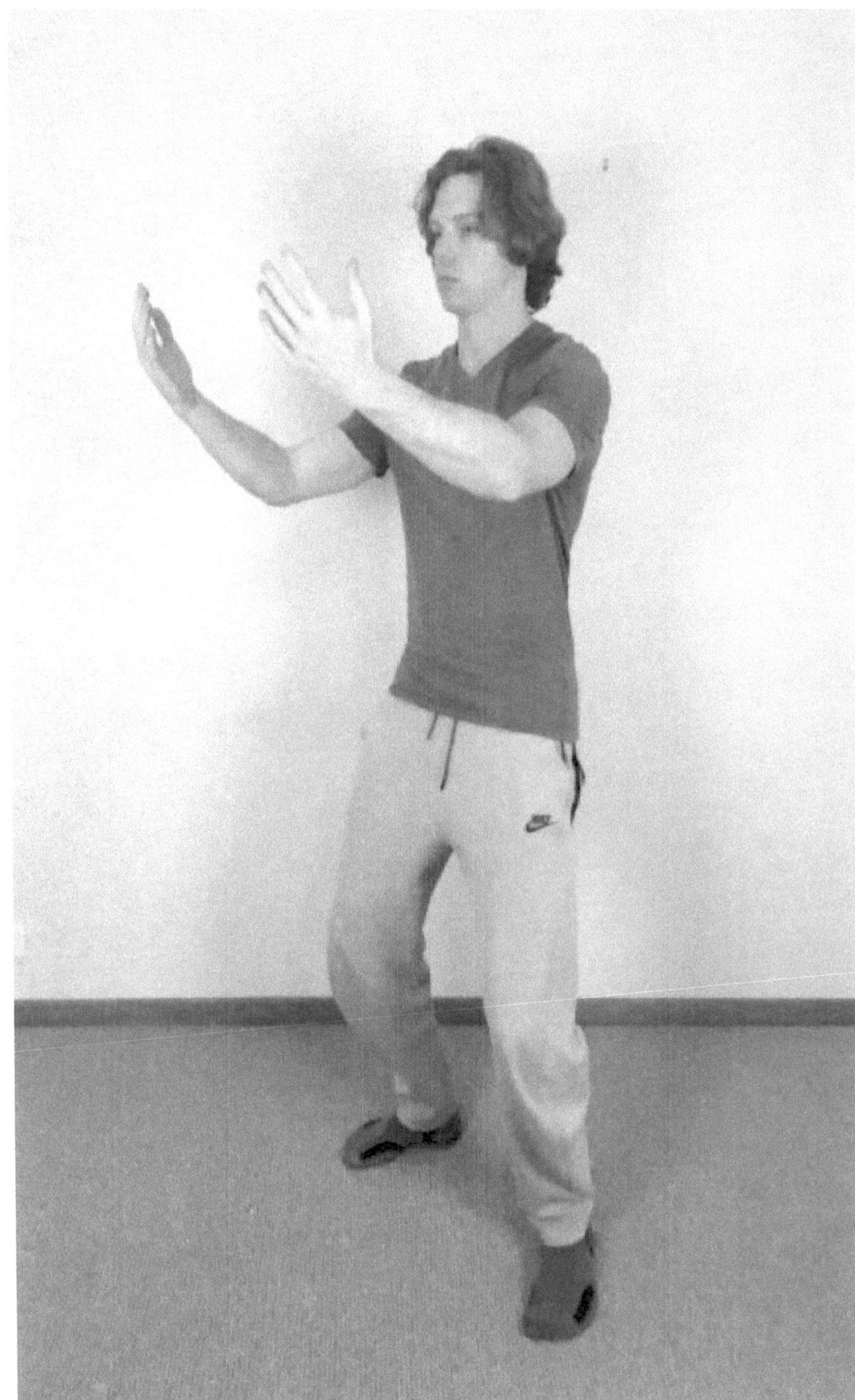

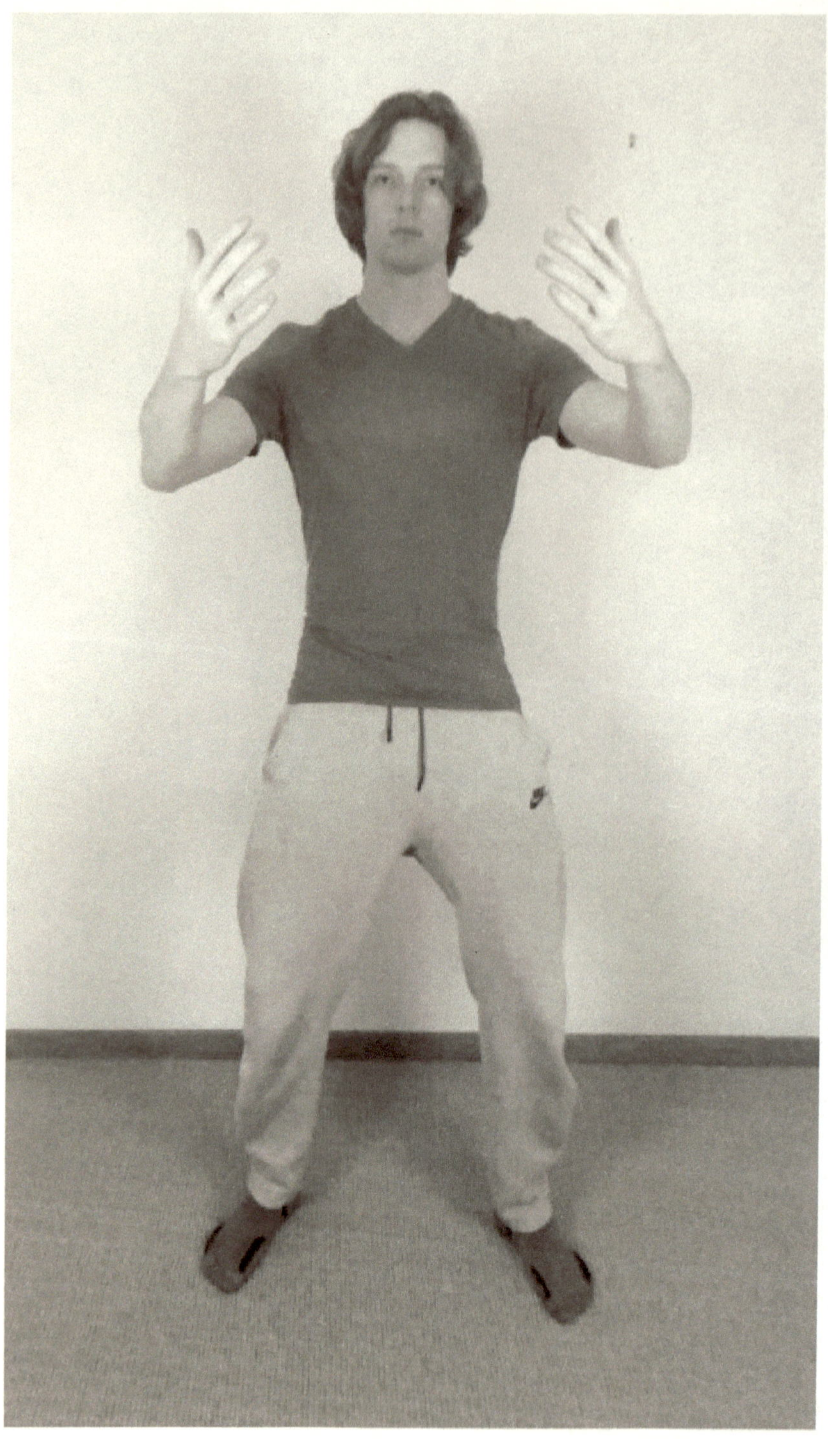

# CHAPTER 3: THE OBSERVATION OF WILHELM REICH

If you are a sufferer of muscular pain, then you stand at a crossroads in your life.

One road has a sign that says, "Purely Physical", and the other has a sign that says "Physical, Emotional and Mental".

Down the "Purely Physical" road, you can choose to take a purely physical approach to muscular pain. You can believe that your chronic muscular pain is not due to your own conscious doing, but due to some physical cause outside of your control. You may continue searching for stretches and strengtheners and other purely physical approaches. You could try injections, surgeries, and all sorts of machines and gadgets.

But know this -- there is nothing down that path of evasion and denial. Nothing but the continued existence of chronic muscular pain. You are more than free to walk that path for as long as you like, and this book will be waiting for you when you are finally ready.

There is an old proverb -- "No matter how far you walk down the wrong path, turn back".

Let's consider the other path.

Down the "Physical, Emotional and Mental" road is a deep exploration of your body, your emotions and your mind. This way is more difficult, but its rewards are great. They include freedom from all chronic muscular pain, emotional wellbeing, and a clear state of mind.

However, down this road you will come face to face with your darkest demons. Every painful emotion that you have ever evaded in your life is waiting for you down this road. So too is every scary thought. To triumph is to understand the nature of all your fear, guilt, regret, anger and so on.

You will understand how chronic muscular pain is the physical manifestation of a complex inner process by which we repress actions, repress emotions and repress thoughts. As you "undo" this process, which you've probably done for decades, you will open the door to great movement, flexibility, coordination, balance, stability, grace and more.

It's also fair to assume that as you triumph down this road, you may further develop your desirable virtues such as rationality, courage, independence, integrity, honesty, justice, productiveness, pride, self-esteem. You may understand yourself better, and how to successfully direct your intentions.

Let's now begin down the road of the "Physical, Emotional and Mental" approach.

We established in the previous chapter:

"When your muscles are chronically tight and painful, it's because you have made a voluntary, conscious choice to hold your muscles in a state of constant tension."

But I don't want you to take my word from that. I want to help you look within, and to know that it is true by reflecting on your own experiences.

Imagine if you were to lie on your back on the floor. You would notice, with enough attention, that you are not completely relaxed onto the floor. Your back may be excessively arched, your knees may be bent, your shoulders may be raised, your hips may be holding your legs inward, and so on.

If you focus on the muscles of your body, you will notice that there is "tension" in your muscles, and it is that tension that is holding your body up off the ground, out of a state of relaxation. This "excess tension" is unnecessary chronic muscular tension that you carry with you at all times, even when you're asleep. It serves no rational purpose. If you focus on the tension, you will almost certainly be aware of the sensation of pain.

Why does this chronic muscular tension and pain exist? The answer to this has been known in the West for almost 100 years, though largely ignored because of its startling implications.

In the 1920s, an Austrian psychoanalyst, named Wilhelm Reich, made a scientific observation that I consider to be the single most important observation regarding chronic muscular tension of the 20th century.

He first observed that any patient who came to him for help with their mind, also possessed a degree of chronic muscular tension, which was often painful. Second, he observed that whenever people would make a breakthrough in their thinking, that is, when they resolve some inner conflict, there would be a simultaneous release of chronic muscular tension. It would vanish, never to return.

This led Reich to conclude that chronic muscular tension is in a 1-to-1 relationship with the inner conflict in one's mind.

This led him to a style of therapy in which he would work simultaneously with the musculature and the mind. He would have patients do special breathing exercises and movements of the spine and pelvis while he conducted therapy.

This flies directly in the face of modern thought on chronic muscular tension, which, as I have already stated, has been unfortunately hijacked by professionals in the fields of "remedial massage", "physiotherapists", "chiropractors", "personal trainers", "yoga teachers" and "calisthenics teachers".

They assert that chronic muscular tension is an issue with the muscles themselves, or the physical structure of the joints and skeleton. They therefore prescribe stretching, strengthening, massage, injections, joint manipulation and so on.

But as you know, these "purely physical approaches" are misguided, because chronic muscular contraction and pain is held in place by instruction from the brain.

Consider this example. Many people have a chronically tense and painful jaw. To treat this, they try all sorts of purely physical solutions. They may wear a special mouthpiece while they sleep. They may have a massage therapist rub their jaw. They may lay down and roll their jaw muscles on a tennis ball or lacrosse ball.

They may see a physiotherapist who says, "It's because you're holding your jaw in the wrong position. You need to hold it over this way. Also, try this stretch and this strengthener." They may go as far as seeing a dentist who reflexively, and with great certainty, recommends surgery to fix the supposedly dysfunctional jaw joint(s).

However, many people have their epiphany about the root cause of muscular pain when I point out that even an extremely tight jaw fully releases at the moment of death. I have witnessed this firsthand. The way completely relaxes and the mouth hangs open. The jaw didn't need to be massaged, or correctly surgically. The constant "contract signals" coming from the brain simply needed to turn off.

**Summary of this chapter:**

- Healing muscular pain requires a commitment to explore your emotions and mind
- Wilhelm Reich observed that solving inner conflicts results in relaxation of muscles
- Purely physical approaches do not address this phenomenon
- Even an extremely tight jaw relaxes completely at the moment of death

**Exercise 3: Balance on One Leg with a Support**

Stand in front of a table or bench (or other suitable piece of furniture), high enough so that you can put your hands on it for support. Then take one leg off the ground. You can hold that leg anywhere you like.

As you balance on one leg, ask yourself, "What would the correct alignment of my body be for this position?" Let go of any images of people you've seen balancing on one leg and go by feeling.

Try to notice any chronically held tensions that are pulling you out of alignment. For example, there may be tensions in your core that are tipping your pelvis forward or back, or to the side.
Search for a configuration of muscular tension that feels efficient, strong,

comfortable, and essentially "better" than your automatic configuration, with which you began the pose.

Play with the angle of hip joint rotation for your standing leg. See how feelings in your body change when you internally or externally rotate your hip joint.

Ask yourself, "Why is my balance not extremely precise? What would need to change in my body and my mind to achieve precise balance?"

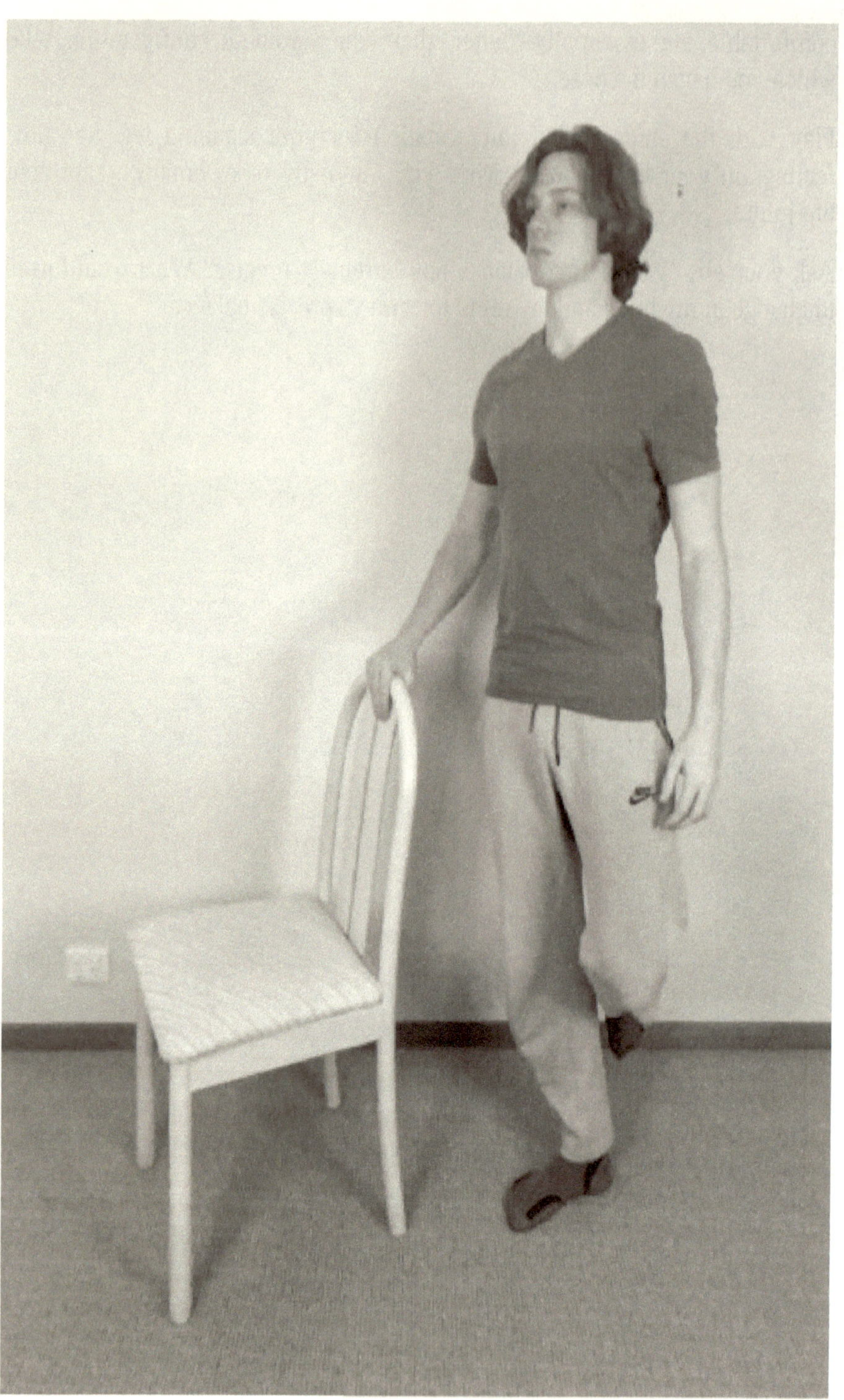

# CHAPTER 4: RELEASING MUSCULAR PAIN EQUALS RELEASING EMOTIONAL PAIN

Why would the brain place a "standing order" for muscles to chronically contract until further notice?

The student of Wilhelm Reich, American Alexander Lowen, made considerable progress in this regard. Lowen points out that "Emotion" is motion. Whenever emotion is experienced, the muscles of the body contract in a certain way. For example, you certainly know that each emotion has a corresponding facial expression. There is also motion throughout the entire body.

Sometimes, emotions can feel awfully bad. Fear, anger, shame, guilt, envy, disappointment, revenge, rage, contempt, regret, disgust, terror, neglect, loneliness, embarrassment, jealousy, grief, and so many more. These can feel so strange and horrible, that we are afraid, even terrified to experience them. And so, we may choose to "hold back" our emotions. How does this "holding back" occur?

Alexander Lowen suggests (as well as I can presently understand) that we hold back emotions by preventing the movement induced in the body with an equal and opposite muscular contraction to essentially "freeze" the emotion. (Note: Lowen does not mention this "equal and opposite" idea. Rather, I inferred it from my knowledge of classical (Newtonian) physics).

Sometimes an emotion may compel us to do something, like yell at someone, or strike them, or to collapse or cry or run away… and we may also counter that action by contracting our muscles to prevent the action.

The freezing of muscles to prevent movement or action, is the physical component of the mind-body process, well known as "repressing emotions". Here are some examples of how tensions in the muscles are associated with repressed emotions.

Repressed fear is often associated with the chronic muscular tensions that bring the body into this closed, protected position, especially muscles of the neck and shoulders, chest and ribs, and inner thighs.

Repressed rage is often associated with chronic tension in the muscles of aggression and punching and kicking, especially the fists, jaw, middle back between the shoulders and legs.

Repressed guilt, regret and sadness are often associated with chronic muscular tensions in the muscles that pull the body out of this "collapsed" body structure and can feel like a weight spread all across the neck, shoulders and back.

Sexual shames, embarrassments, inadequacies and disgusts often lead to chronic muscular tensions in the hips, pelvic floor and lower abs…

And all that is just the tip of the iceberg.

Because literally any time in your life that you have repressed an emotion, and not later allowed it to be fully experienced, you have induced a chronic muscular tension into the body by contracting muscles to prevent the action or movement that the emotion is trying to perform.

Any person with chronic muscular pain is probably wise to assume that there are thousands, probably tens of thousands of unresolved physical, emotional and mental conflicts that all collectively contribute to their experience of pain.

The total chronic muscular tension in your body, is thus a summation of all the muscular tension that is being constantly held to prevent unwanted emotions from expressing.

Therefore, the way toward solving chronic muscular tension is about "letting go" of the contractions designated to repress emotions and experiencing those emotions. Those two activities are one in the same. Letting go of chronic muscular tension is equal to experiencing repressed emotions.

That's quite important, so I'll say it again -- letting go of chronic muscular tension is equal to experiencing repressed emotions.

The next question to be answered is therefore: "How does someone experience their repressed emotions?"

Just before we delve into that, I need to cover a common objection.

Many people have pain that clearly stems from injuries. A fall involving a twisting of the spine, or the hyperextension of a joint, or the pulling of a muscle, tendon or ligament.

Is this covered by what I refer to as "repressed emotions".

Yes. The emotion is "fear". In the case of such injuries, it is fear of reinjury, and top of that, fear of movement. A person who is injured puts in place many chronic contractions of their muscle, out of fear of moving in a way that could aggravate their injury.

Often a simple sprain or pull can lead to layers upon layers of muscular tension all throughout the body. To recover from this, the person will eventually have to calmly repeat the exact positions and movements that they have been avoiding. When they do so, they will experience extreme amounts of fear, which has been lurking within.

Tissue of the body heals with time, but inhibition of emotion and movement causes chronic pain forever. To release pain, a person must face the exact movement or emotion that they've been avoiding.

It almost sounds as if I'm suggesting that the method to release chronic muscular pain is "therapy". But I'm not. Therapy can help a person get a semi-logical understanding of their problems in life, and help them "cope", but only very rarely will it have the effect of releasing chronic muscular tension.

And by the insight of Wilhelm Reich, if there is no release of chronic muscular tension, there is no release of repressed emotion, and there is no true resolution of inner conflict.

The solution to all of this is a type of activity that incorporates your muscles, your emotions and your thoughts.

So far, I have not touched on "thoughts". I have only said "emotions". I am saving the discussion of thoughts for later because it's the most complex. You will soon see that it's not really "repressed emotions", but "repressed thought", at the center of all this. Though perhaps the term "evaded thought", is more accurate.

**Summary of this chapter:**

- We can "hold back" emotions by squeezing our muscles
- Every single repressed emotion is guarded by chronic muscular tension
- Fear is involved with every chronic muscular tension
- A solution that simultaneously considers physical, emotional and mental factors is required

**Exercise 4: Lean Backward and Tip the Head Backward**

This exercise should be done slowly, with care.

Leaning backward or tipping the head backward, causing the spine to "extend", usually generates significant discomfort in the lower back or neck. The muscles around the vertebrae reactively squeeze extremely hard. People generally will not tolerate this experience for very long. In general, people entirely avoid leaning back or tipping their head back.

This exercise is not in itself dangerous or uncomfortable. The vertebrae of the spine are completely capable of moving this way. Consider a "back bridge" in yoga -- people who can do this do not have a "special" spine.

The reason we may experience extreme tightening or pain when leaning back, or tipping the head back, is because we have dissociated from the muscles of the spine. We have lost the ability to perceive them or control them, because we have repressed the negative emotions that are "trapped" in those muscles.

Over the years, you should learn to lean backward, and tip your head backward. Though this will not be a fast process. You will need to do it gradually.

Today, either stand, kneel or sit, and lean backward and tip your head back slightly. You may wish to hold the pose for a minute or two. Notice the uncomfortable tensions and ask "What is that tension? Why does it exist?" Promise yourself that you will eventually find out and release the tensions.

Note: You may open your jaw, or keep it closed. Both are different experiences.

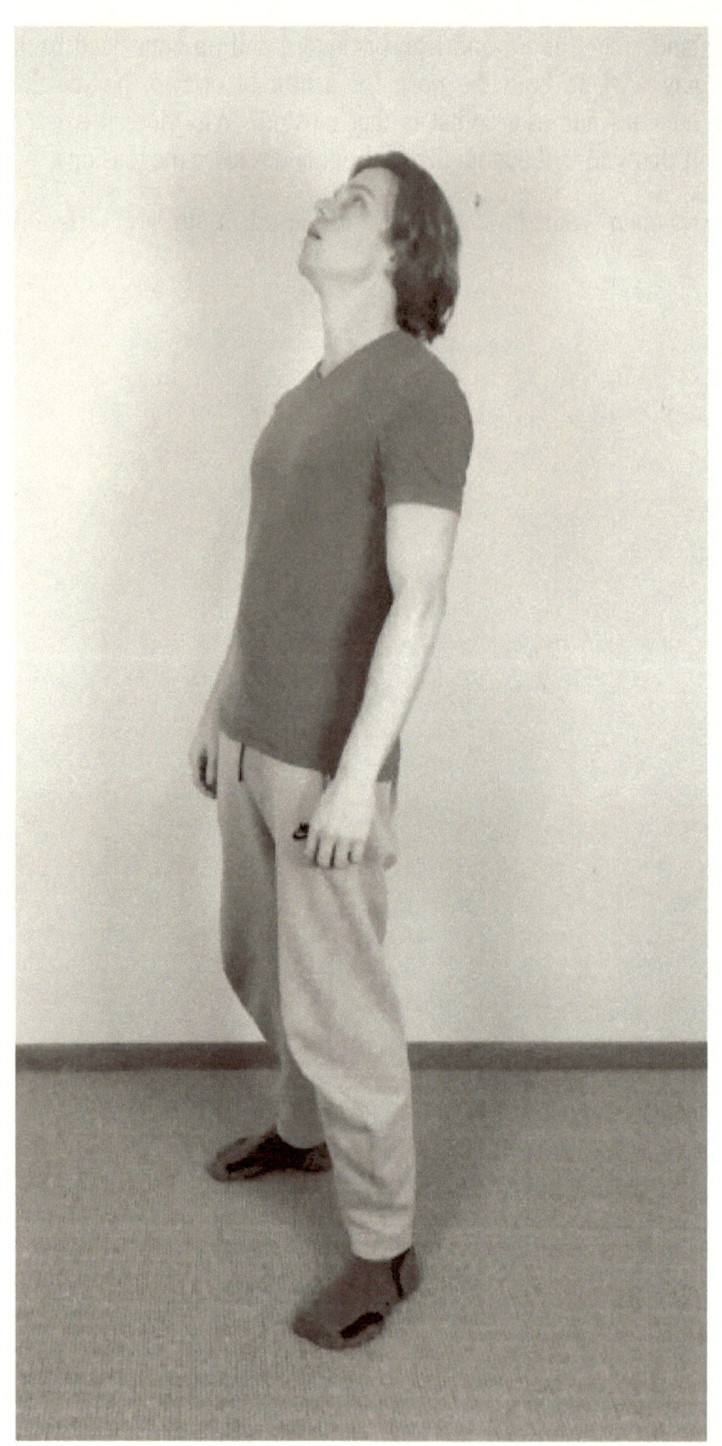

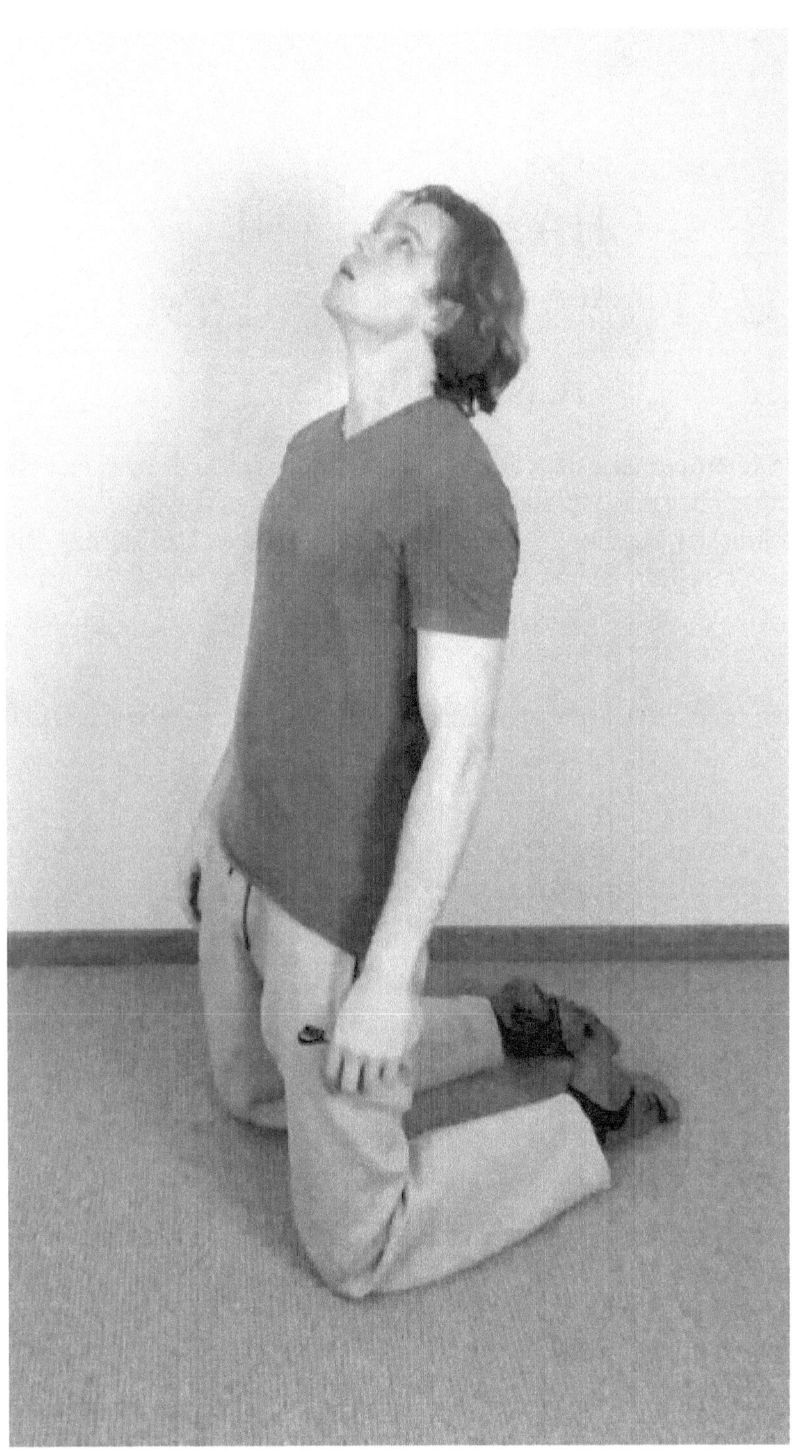

# CHAPTER 5: THE GATEWAY TO REPRESSED EMOTIONS

I will share my personal story of how I discovered a method that incorporates physical, emotional and mental factors. In a way, I am torn about whether to include it or not, because I consider this book to be a work of science. Did Einstein tell the story of how he formulated his model of relativity, or did he just present the model? Of course, he just presented it, because mathematics, as a science, requires no historical or aesthetic support.

However, people frequently tell me that they can relate to my story, and find it quite useful, so I've chosen to include it.

I first noticed that I had pain in my body at age 18 when I was in my first year of University, studying Aeronautical Engineering. My neck, shoulders and forearms would ache whenever I used a computer or wrote with a pen. My low back would ache whenever I sat in a chair. My knees began to ache at the gym.

Soon standing in one place for too long or walking hurt, and eventually it just hurt all the time. I tried every single mainstream physical treatment method you've ever heard of. I stretched, I did yoga, I got regular massages. I learned good posture, and people even said I had great posture. I saw chiropractors for spinal adjustments, and radiologists for injections.

But there were no pleasing results. And believe me, I was extremely dedicated. Seeing as other people studied just as much as me, lifted weights just as much as me, and generally had equal or worse posture and form to me, I thought the pain was because I was "somehow using my muscles incorrectly".

I didn't just have physical pain, I also had a lot of anger, anxiety, guilt, sadness and regret. I sought to feel better in classic self-development books like "How to Win Friends and Influence People", "7 Habits of Highly Effective People", "Awaken the Giant Within", "Think and Grow Rich". I learned public speaking at Toastmasters. I learned to be "confident" and sociable. I "felt the fear and did it anyway". I sought "success".

I received 1st Class Honors in my degree. I worked first in Engineering, and later in Corporate Finance. I ran an online business and earned over USD $10,000 per month. I travelled to 40 countries. But I still had physical pain everywhere in my body, worse all the time. Truly intolerable, insufferable pain. And I was still constantly anxious, angry, sad, guilty and regretful. About what, who knows? Just a thick fog of these undifferentiated feelings, from unknown sources.

"Lifestyle" is great, but it does not even begin to compare to a good feeling body, healthy emotions and a calm mind.

I suppose the only thing that kept me together was hope. Hope that I would one day reach a day when I would begin to figure it all out, fix everything and feel good. For you, I hope that day is the day you began reading this book.

For me, it came suddenly on a day after 12 long years of body-wide pain. Better late than never, right? It was a day in August 2017, living in Medellin, Colombia. A day like any other day in The City of Eternal Spring when I stumbled on my first hint.

I found a YouTube channel by a Finnish mobility Expert, Eero Westerberg. He moved so well, and the way he explained it… was like no one had ever explained movement before. All about "feeling the muscles" and paying attention to sensations in your muscles during exercises, rather than the external visual appearance or "form" of the exercise.

I hired him to Coach me, and I learned all about the mind-muscle connection, not just the facts, but how to use it. How to awaken my dormant "muscle sense", which is indeed a real thing that scientists call "Proprioception", meaning "Self-perception", the neurological ability to perceive your own body. I was getting a literally world class education in how to move my body.

I learned to control the level of tension in my muscles as I did exercise. I learned to move with smooth control and stability. I got in touch with muscles I didn't even know existed and learned to move my joints in ways I didn't know they moved. And I began to notice that my body was indeed feeling a bit better. But nothing could have prepared me for what happened next.

I was trying all sorts of different movements, now that I was being educated on how to move my body, and one day I looked up a term called "developmental movement", because I was suspicious that what I needed to do was really, really easy movement - movement so slow and easy, that I'd never taken the time to do, as I'd been living in a "rush" all my life.

So up came a video by a woman named Alicia Patterson, teaching one exercise from a group of developmental movements from decades ago called Bartenieff Fundamentals.

Alicia warned that doing these movements could trigger repressed emotions to release. At the time I was like, "Well that's not a real thing, but I'll try it anyway". I was blown away.

Sure enough, as I did the exercise, moving back and forth, rocking, slowly and consciously as I learned from Eero, paying close attention to the sensations coming from my muscles, suddenly something happened. A feeling of fear... a clear feeling of tension in my lower back... confusion... and suddenly a flashback to some distressed emotional moment in childhood.

And just like that, a tension in my lower back released. It simply turned off. A painful emotion experienced and resolved, with a simultaneous release of chronic muscular tension.

I was eager to repeat the experience! Unfortunately, none of exercises on Alicia's channel had a similar effect.

I looked up videos of the other Bartenieff Fundamentals exercises on other YouTube channels. I tried them, but I didn't get a similar result.

Had I just gotten lucky? I wasn't sure, but even that single experience, I was immediately certain in that moment of 3 things, 1) That chronic muscular tension was a mind-body phenomenon. 2) That slow movement with deep focus on muscles could help release trapped negative emotions. 3) That trapped negative emotions were somehow linked with chronic muscular tension.

And so, I began to experiment on my own. Trial and error. Whenever I had a moment of free time, I was trying different movements, trying to trigger the same experience. And I probably would not be talking to you today, had I not had tremendous success.

In a mere 10 days, I was able to replicate the experience approximately 100 times. And I noticed a clear pattern. Each experience started with exceedingly small back and forth movements of a joint, signifying turning muscles on and off.

These movements would help me to deeply focus on a specific tension in a muscle (or muscle group, if the tension covered a wide area).

Suddenly, there would be an onset of fear or confusion, followed by a flashback and an experience of a trapped negative emotion, followed ultimately by the release of a chronic muscular tension.

I was over the moon. A couple of the best things, after just those 10 days, were that I longer needed to use a "back rest" whenever I sat down to work… and I no longer needed to wear special wrist braces on both hands to prevent pain while typing. And just in general, so many muscles all over my body felt so, so much better.

If that were all I achieved, that would have been enough for me. Though I'd had a taste of what was possible, and I wanted more. I sensed that it was probably possible to completely cure all chronic muscular tension from my body.

**Summary of this chapter:**

- I had physical pain all over my body
- I spent 12 years trying purely physical approaches
- The 1st breakthrough came from learning to "perceive" my

muscles
- The 2nd breakthrough was finding a gateway to repressed emotions via small, slow, focused movements

## Exercise 5: Lift Your Head Up Off the Floor

Lay either on your stomach or your back. Take as long as you like to get comfortable and present. Check for any muscular tension that you can "turn off" and do so.

Raise your head so that its weight is no longer resting on the floor, but contact is still being made. If you're on your stomach, then just the skin of your forehead should be touching. If you're on your back, then just the back of your head should touch (through your hair).

Hold this position for an extended period of time and observe the configuration of muscular tension you are using. Undoubtedly, you are overly tense, because you are not only lifting your head up, you are also fighting all the chronic muscular tension that is working against you.

What is this chronic muscular tension? Where is it? Is it in your throat? The back of your neck? Your shoulders? Your chest? Your ribs? Your lower back? Your hips? Your legs?

Pay attention to all the tension in your body and try to feel it. Ask yourself what you feel, and why you feel it.

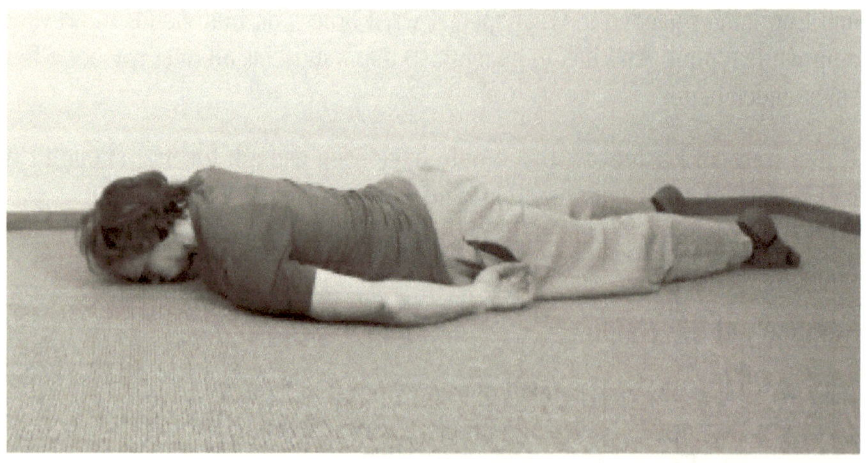

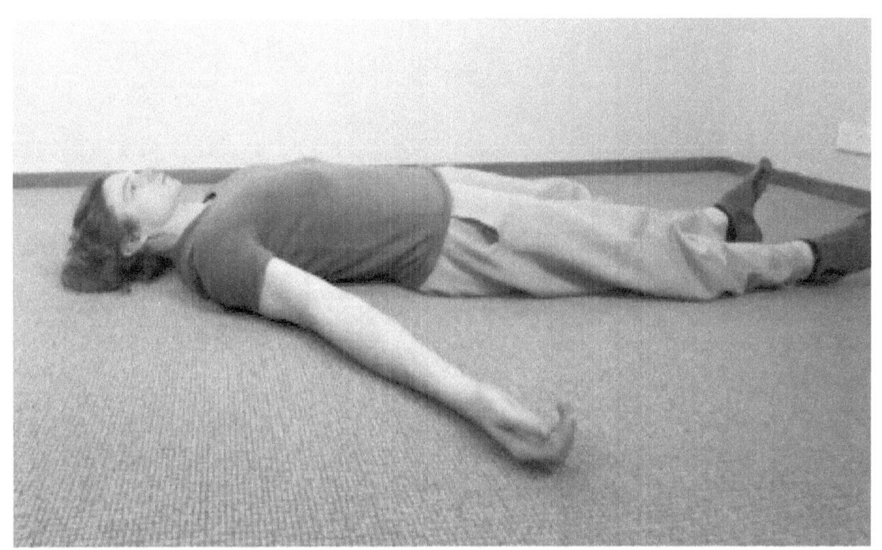

# CHAPTER 6: THE EVASION OF THOUGHT

Having taken the first step, I wanted to go all the way. At this point, as I write this book, it seems to me that I've gone most of the way. So much pain has disappeared from my body. My emotions are much calmer and healthier, and my mind is sharper, more focused and more intentful.

To do this, I had to take actions that caused the release of painful tension from my life. But how can one figure out which actions to take? The answer is to accumulate knowledge of the body, emotions and mind. With knowledge, you have information that can serve as a basis for your conscious choices.

On one front, I read hundreds of scientific papers about neurology, anatomy and muscle function.

On a second front, I took up martial arts, gymnastics and ballet, and continued movement training with Eero. I also did a week-long intensive training course with a movement instructor named Egwin Ertl.

On a third front, I began to devour the most complex philosophical, psychoanalytical and mind-body scientific works of the 20th century. Objectivism by Ayn Rand, Dianetics by Hubbard, Character Analysis by Wilhelm Reich, Bioenergetics by Alexander Lowen.

As my knowledge of the body, emotions and mind grew, my ability to understand myself grew, and I became able to resolve even the most complex pains and emotions grew.

I "triggered my brain" to release many chronic muscular tensions out of my body, with simultaneous experience of repressed painful emotions.

Here are some examples, which you can probably relate to:

- Shock and trauma from past injuries
- Fear of positions or movements that I thought could cause pain or injury.
- Hatred, rage, revenge toward people who I felt had wronged me.
- Grief over the loss of property, virtues and loved ones.
- Embarrassment and shame about public humiliations.
- Frustration and resentment toward society as a whole.
- Envy toward those who had what I thought they didn't deserve.
- Disappointment about life not following my rigid and unrealistic expectations.
- Guilt over every single act that violated my own morality. Unearned guilt over acts that violated the morality of others.
- Fear of being beaten, fear of going insane, fear of being murdered, fear of suicide.
- Terror from people legitimately threatening my life.
- Scary thoughts about the nature of the Universe and my role in it. Whether life is worth living or not.
- Self-doubt, romantic jealousies, sensual disgusts.

Every single emotional experience that ever happened and wasn't fully processed was "still there". Blocked by chronic muscular tension.

I have probably experienced over 10,000 unique releases of chronic tension. Indeed, that means that there were over 10,000 unique painful emotions trapped within me. It may be like this for you too, but don't let that daunt you -- it only means there is huge potential for positive change.

When you observe something happening over 10,000 times, you certainly notice patterns.

Every time a negative emotion would process, and a chronic muscular tension would release, I would also observe that there was some particular "thought" wrapped up in the tension. Some irrationality, or confusion, or conflict. Some "false belief". Some incorrect "conviction" that I'd chosen to believe because the truth was too painful to contemplate.

I began to suspect that it wasn't "emotions" I'd been evading, it was thought. Thought about things that were too confrontational or too confusing. Because I couldn't deal with their implications. Because I preferred to live in denial than face reality.

I didn't come to this suspicion without assistance. I suspected that thoughts had "something to do with it" … but I couldn't put all the pieces together until I read this quote by Ayn Rand:

"Thinking is man's only basic virtue, from which all the others proceed. And his basic vice, the source of all his evils, is that nameless act which all of you practice, but struggle never to admit: the act of blanking out, the willful suspension of one's consciousness, the refusal to think—not blindness, but the refusal to see; not ignorance, but the refusal to know. It is the act of unfocusing your mind and inducing an inner fog to escape the responsibility of judgment—on the unstated premise that a thing will not exist if only you refuse to identify it, that A will not be A so long as you do not pronounce the verdict "It is." Non-thinking is an act of annihilation, a wish to negate existence, an attempt to wipe out reality. But existence exists; reality is not to be wiped out, it will merely wipe out the wiper. By refusing to say "It is," you are refusing to say "I am." By suspending your judgment, you are negating your person. When a man declares: "Who am I to know?" he is declaring: "Who am I to live?""

Here we have the greatest philosophical mind of all time declaring that evading thoughts is the "source of all evils", and I was also noticing that behind every painful muscular tension, behind every painful repressed emotion, was thought that I'd been evading.

At first, I played with the idea that possibly "evasion of thoughts" is the root cause of pain. But eventually I decided that "evasion of thoughts" simply "goes with" pain. There are things which are so much more primary to life, such as awareness, focus, perception. These precede conceptual thought.

However, the realization that pain generally involves some level of thought evasion, implied that a generalized method for releasing pain should help guide us toward thoughts we have been evading. When we come face to face with previously evaded thoughts, we are surprised to learn that such a thought was in our mind.

That's because we have hidden them well and covered up any traces of their existence. We have buried them deep, and yet they remain as faulty, unquestioned premises that form our character and guide our actions in every moment of our lives.

Until we access and resolve these evaded thoughts, we will be in fear of those thoughts, we will feel the painful emotions that those thoughts are generating, and our actions will be guided according to them.

**Summary of this chapter:**

- Knowledge of the body, emotions and mind is crucial for healing pain
- Every experience in which you didn't fully process a painful emotion is "trapped inside you"
- Evasion of thoughts is deeply tied with repression and therefore chronic muscular pain
- A method that heals chronic muscular pain should help us find and confront our evaded thoughts

**Exercise 6: Hold Arms Above You with Shoulders Shrugged**

The muscles that "raise" the shoulders usually have a lot of chronic muscular tension. We are often trying to "relax" our shoulder muscles when what we really need to do is feel them to the fullest extent.

Raise your arms to vertical above your head, and then shrug your shoulders upward for extra height. If you can't get to the vertical, an angle is fine. Modifications to make these exercises as easy as they need to be are generally a good thing.

Hold this position for an extended period of time, stopping only when you become bored or "can't take it anymore".

While you hold the position, investigate your shoulder muscles. Figure out how they work, and which chronic tensions are in play. See if you become aware of any emotions, fears or thoughts while in the position. Ask yourself "What's that about?"

You are welcome to occasionally lower and raise your shoulders, or even do some circular motions. Anything goes, as long as you're investigating.

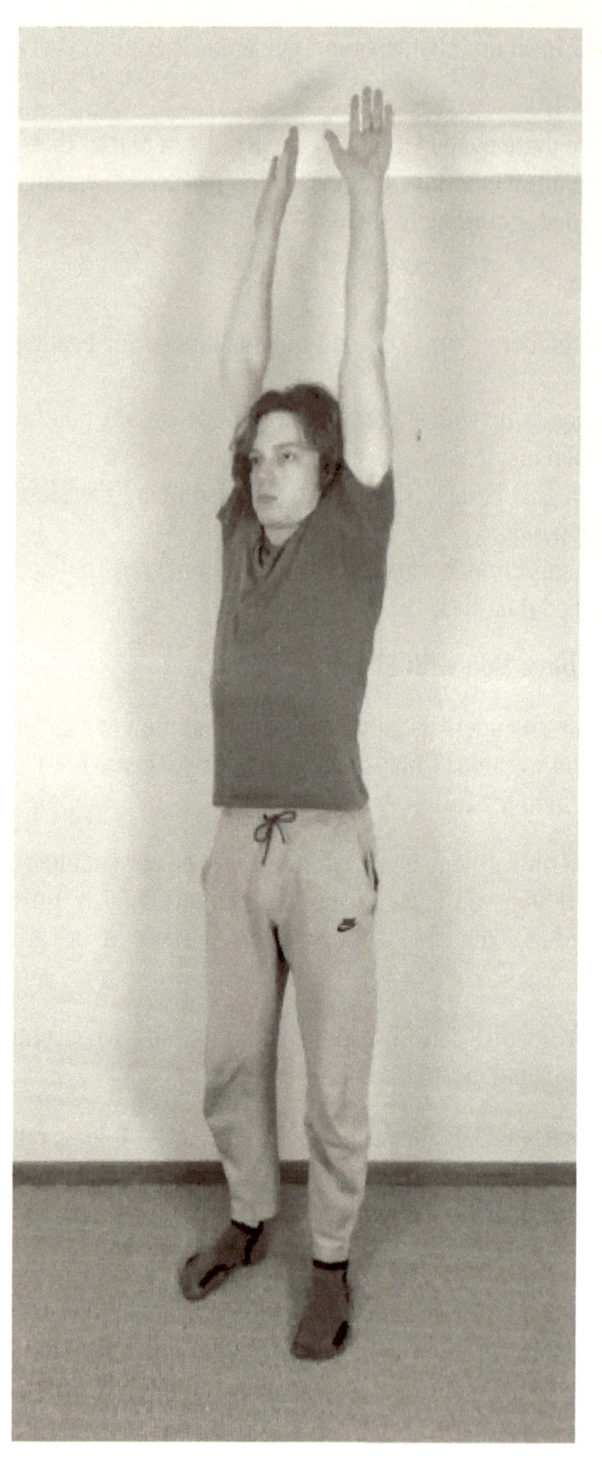

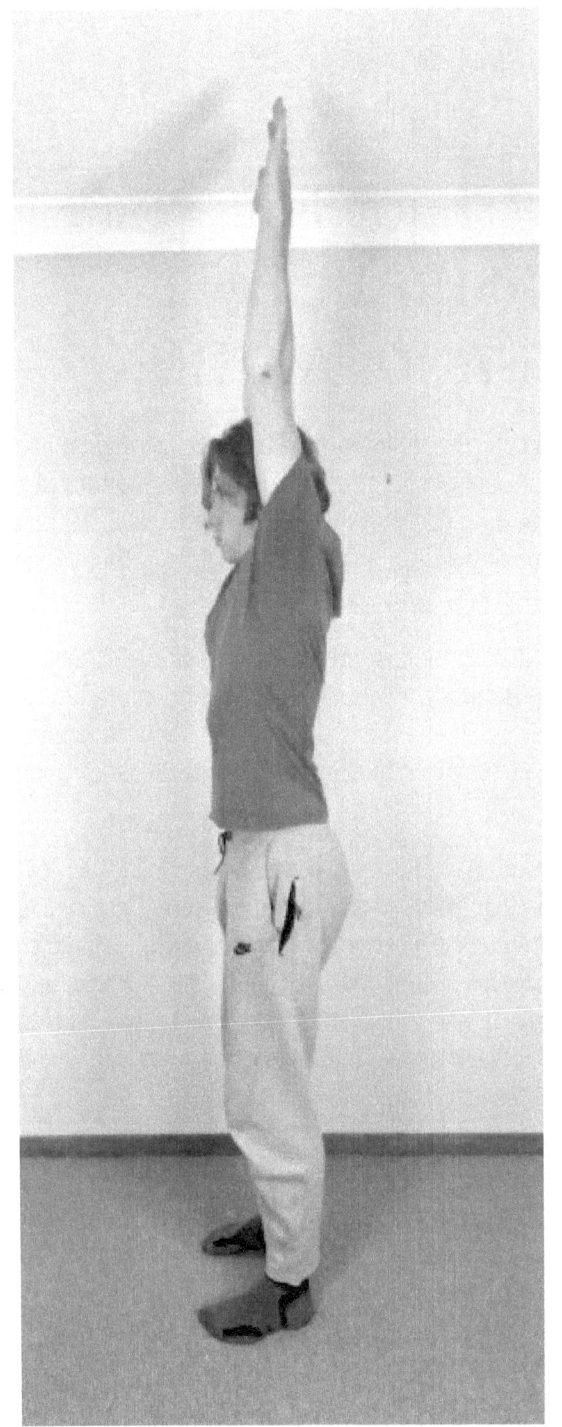

# CHAPTER 7: THE RELATIONSHIP BETWEEN THOUGHT AND EMOTION

To progress, we must establish the relationship between thoughts and emotions. The great myth of emotions in society is that emotions are automatically generated by sensation. That simply seeing something, hearing something, being exposed to something, will automatically generate an instinctive emotion that is beyond your conscious control.

However, it can be shown that emotions are not automatic, instinctual responses to external stimuli. Rather, thoughts precede emotions, and that emotions are physical reactions, consequential to a person's thoughts. Specifically, their preconceived premises and inferences made based upon these premises.

At the sight of a dog, one person may feel fear, while another may feel joy. The aroma of a freshly baked cake may cause one person to feel desire and anticipation, while another is reminded of their aunt, passed away, who once baked that same cake, and thus feels the sorrow of their loss. Choose any situation and you will quickly think of circumstances where one person would feel one emotion, and another person would feel a completely different emotion, in response to the exact same stimuli.

Let us consult Ayn Rand for the reasons behind this:

"Just as the pleasure-pain mechanism of man's body is an automatic indicator of his body's welfare or injury, a barometer of its basic alternative, life or death—so the emotional mechanism of man's consciousness is geared to perform the same function, as a barometer that registers the same alternative by means of two basic emotions: joy or suffering. Emotions are the automatic results of man's value judgments integrated by his subconscious; emotions are estimates of that which furthers man's values or threatens them, that which is for him or against him—lightning calculators giving him the sum of his profit or loss.

But while the standard of value operating the physical pleasure-pain mechanism of man's body is automatic and innate, determined by the nature of his body—the standard of value operating his emotional mechanism, is not. Since man has no automatic knowledge, he can have no automatic values; since he has no innate ideas, he can have no innate value judgments.

Man is born with an emotional mechanism, just as he is born with a cognitive mechanism; but, at birth, both are "tabula rasa." It is man's cognitive faculty, his mind, that determines the content of both. Man's emotional mechanism is like an electronic computer, which his mind has to program—and the programming consists of the values his mind chooses.

But since the work of man's mind is not automatic, his values, like all his premises, are the product either of his thinking or of his evasions: man chooses his values by a conscious process of thought—or accepts them by default, by subconscious associations, on faith, on someone's authority, by some form of social osmosis or blind imitation. Emotions are produced by man's premises, held consciously or subconsciously, explicitly or implicitly."

From The Virtue of Selfishness, 1964, by Ayn Rand.

Whenever something we value is lost, taken, threatened, damaged, etc, we feel a negative emotion. Also, whenever our chance of obtaining or achieving something we value is diminished, we will also feel a negative emotion.

Something of value could be our status, our reputation, our job, our money, our property, our liberty, our happiness, our rights, our life, our family, our friends, our community, our country, our species. Negative emotions in response to a perceived threat to these values come in different flavors - raw fear, rage, shame, sadness, guilt, grief, envy, embarrassment, and so on.

There is absolutely nothing wrong with feeling emotions. Both positive and negative emotions are to be expected in life. Life is saturated with ups and downs that frequently cause emotional reactions. This is all perfectly fine.

The important thing to accept is that it is our thoughts that determine our emotional responses. Without thought, there is no emotion. Even a baby's crying is because the baby has consciously formed such premises as: "Mum's attention good", "Being alone bad", "Drinking milk good", "Hungry bad", or "Warm good", "Cold bad", "Comfort good", "Pain bad".

And therefore, behind every repressed emotion, is one or premises about what is valuable and what is true. These premises determine our "gut reactions" to events.

You could consider the set of all your premises (every single one of them) to be what is generally referred to as a "belief system".

If our premises about ourselves, others, reality, life and so on, reflect an attitude and character of rationality, independence, pride, self-esteem and honour, then our emotional responses will be rational, and not particularly uncomfortable. We will be able to easily handle each event as it comes along, and we will not be excessively "damaged" by it.

If however, our premises about ourselves, others, reality, life and so on, reflect an attitude and character of weakness, deception, self-doubt, self-loathing, low self-esteem, insecurity, and so one, then our emotional responses will be chaotic, heavy, painful, confusing, scary and so on. We will feel like something very bad is happening to us, and that our life is becoming much worse.

Furthermore, we will lack a view of life that lets us interpret emotionally charged events objectively. We will be literally unable to perceive, consider, analyze or become conscious events. We will not be able to end the pain, because we are unable to make sense of it. We are unable to understand, objectively, why "everything is OK" in spite of what happened.

Emotionally charged "painful moments" will haunt us with physically perceived emotional pain until we gain the "intellectual" strength to look at them objectively and realize, truthfully that "everything is OK". Intellectual strength is not the ability to do math or science or have good grammar -- it is ability to comprehend reality objectively.

Consider a character who holds firm convictions that their mind is capable of thinking, that they are worthy of living, that they probably can deal most of that which life could throw at them. This is the character of rationality and self-esteem.

Now consider a character who is uncertain about everything. They're not sure if reality really exists, or if it's just an illusion playing before their consciousness. They're not sure if they have free will, or everything is predetermined. They're not really sure why they have value, or if they deserve to be alive. This is the character of severely limited self-esteem.

The first character has superior intellectual strength and will therefore be able to process emotional pain easily. The second will be unable to make sense of emotional pain. They will have reactions such as "why is this happening to me?" ... "it's not fair" ... "who do I blame for this?" ... "This is all so terrible and unfortunate" ... "somebody do something about this" ... "how could I ever possibly feel better".

As we build our intellectual strength, that is build our rationality, independence, pride, self-esteem and others, we build our ability to deal with past painful events objectively, resolve them, integrate them and transcend them.

Thus, there is a lot of objective thought to be done, to resolve pain.

**Summary of this chapter:**

- Emotions are lightning-quick responses determined by the content of our mind
- Characters of high "intellectual strength" can handle painful emotions
- Self-esteem is a large component of intellectual strength
- A large amount of objective thought must be done to resolve pain

**Exercise 7: Fingertips on the Ground**

Most people complain about "tight hamstrings" and a "tight lower back". Certainly, these are two of the most common reasons for which people see a physiotherapist, who is more than delighted to offer "stretches". They love stretches because it provides an immediate illusion of a result.

The following exercise is not a stretch. It is intended to help you experience your entire body in a complex position. If you have in your mind that you're stretching while you do this exercise, you will not achieve results. Let go of that intention.

Bend down and place your fingertips on the floor. Your feet may be in any position whatsoever. You may move your fingertips to any location whatsoever.

There is an ideal situation in which your legs are perfectly straight, your body is curled down close to your legs, and your hands easily touch the floor, though that is a distant outcome, which you need not consider right now. All you have to do is maintain your fingertips touching the floor.

Feel your legs, feel your back, feel your neck, feel your core. Search for inhibitions in your movement patterns, and "rules" you have for your body that keep you in an uncomfortable position. In general, you should move out of discomfort and into more comfort at all times.

Some shaking may occur, and that is fine. Go through it. Maybe even enjoy it.

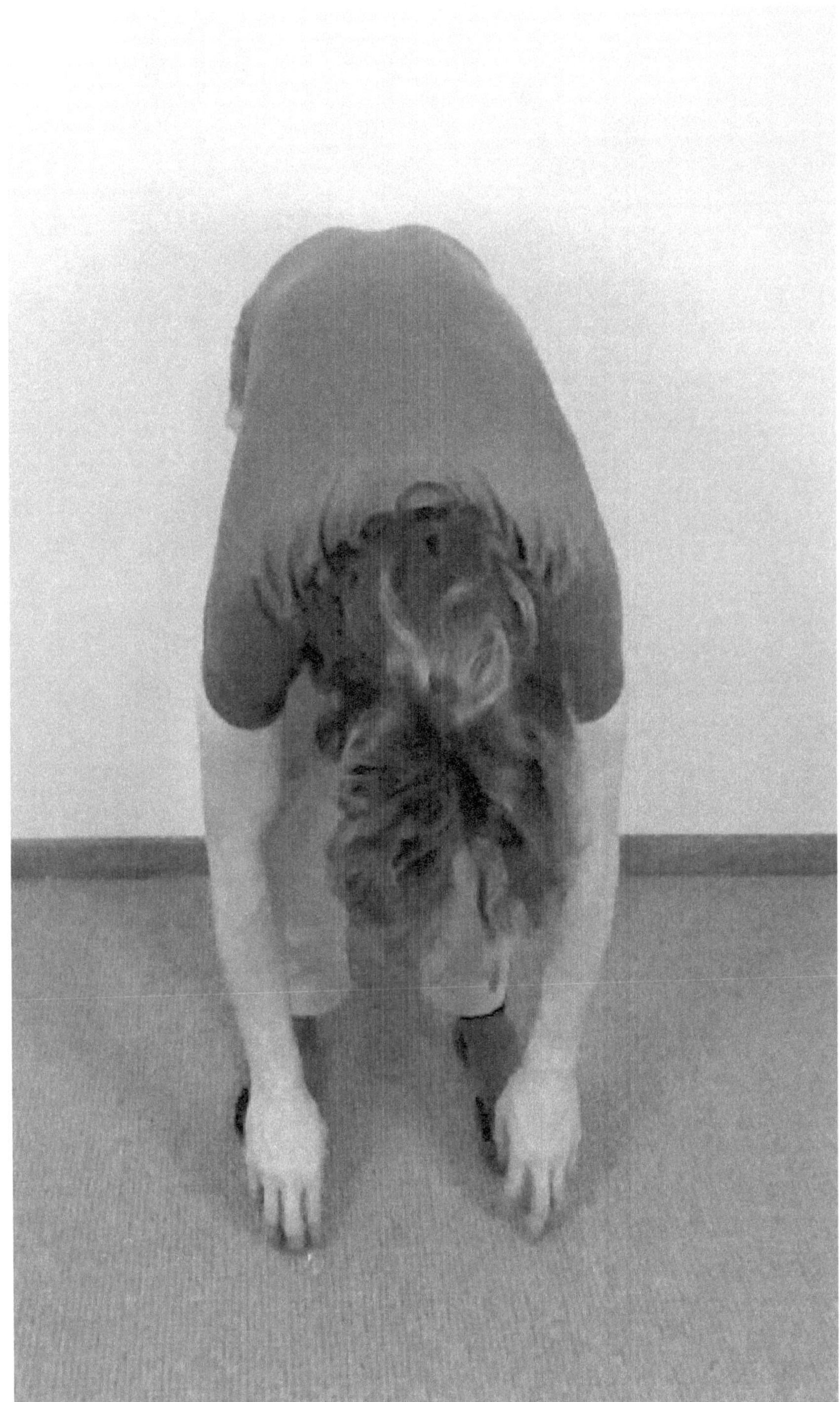

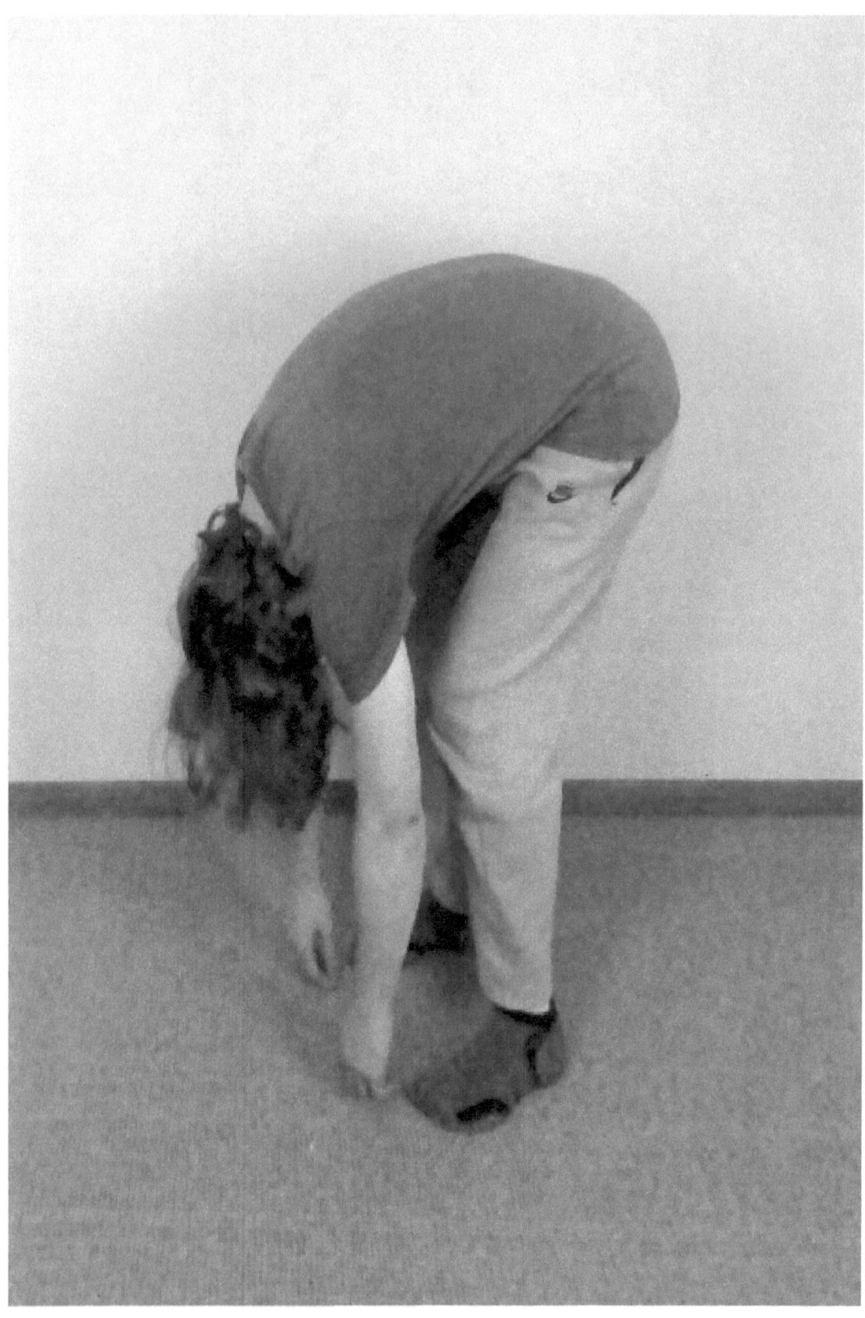

# CHAPTER 8: MIND BODY PAIN UNITS

We have covered much of the relationship between the physical, the emotional and the mental realms. We have established that we voluntarily choose to squeeze our muscles to prevent the activation of painful emotions. That is to say, figuratively, that we are "pushing back against" the intention that the emotion is trying to cause or express. We also established that emotions are governed by our thoughts.

Let's introduce an abstract example for consideration, so that we can see how this works. A betrayal. Someone you trust betrays you. It could be a friend, a lover, a family member. Someone you trusted very much and would never expect to betray you.

If you lack the intellectual strength to deal with this, then possessed by mental confusion and overwhelm, and you will have no means to escape this state. Remember, intellectual strength is an "all encompassing" measure of such virtues as self-esteem, rationality, pride, independence, objectivity.

Let's assume that it is indeed the case that you lack the intellectual strength to deal with this betrayal. Mentally, you are confused and overwhelmed. Emotionally, you feel multiple negative emotions. Physically, your muscles clench.

You now have two choices. To become conscious of the betrayal, or to evade it. "Becoming conscious" of the experience is neither immediate nor automatic. We must actively perceive it, observe it, analyse it, make sense of it, understand it, integrate it, transcend it.

This process of "becoming conscious", runs parallel to "feeling the emotion", and therefore "feeling the pain". Therefore, to become conscious of our experiences, we must feel the pain of our experiences. To become conscious of our lives (and of reality), we must feel all the pain of our lives. There is no shortcut, and no way around it.

Until you "become conscious" of this betrayal, that is to say "work through the experience and come to relate with it on objective, non-attached terms", you will continue to be tormented by the negative emotions, and you will feel the squeeze of the muscles. Your muscles will not relax, and you will retain a measure of anxiety, confusion and disclarity.

If we lack the capacity to reason our way through to total consciousness of an experience, which implies that we are simultaneously too afraid of the pain that it comes with, then we may choose to "evade" this experience. During "evasion", we do multiple things.

Physically, we will introduce a "counter tension" that prevents the expression of the emotion. Perceptually, we block off feeling so that we can't detect the tension, or the emotion. Mentally, we evade thinking. In total, what we are doing is evading reality itself.

We try to erase entire slices of reality that carry painful emotion. We block them from our memory. We block them from our analytical mind. We block them from our perception.

After doing this for a long time, the pain essentially is "overflowing", and even though we're already squeezing our muscles hard, we've reached full capacity, and reach a point where we "can't deal with anything anymore". Different pains are constantly being "triggered", causing us to describe ourselves as "anxious", "stressed", "depressed" or having chronic guilt or regret.

Frequent evasion leads us to live life as if we were navigating through a web of tangled thorns, constantly cutting ourselves every time we make a slightly wrong move, with the constant fear that we might accidentally trip and fall into a world of agony. But what we really need to do, is stop evading the thorns, and instead take out the shearers and deal with these thorns once and for all.

If you have a lot of pain in your life, I think that the best thing you can do is consider that big amorphous blob of undifferentiated pain to be simply a "summation" of thousands of unique pains. This is much less daunting than an unidentified, shapeless force.

I came up with a name for these thousands (which could be tens of thousands, hundreds of thousands, or even millions) of pains: Mind Body Pain Unit.

Anywhere in your body where you experience chronic pain, there are almost certainly many Mind-Body Pain Units in operation.

Each Mind-Body Pain Unit has the following features:

- A chronic muscular tension
- A physical pain
- A blocked emotion
- A fear of that emotion
- A corresponding moment in your past
- A blocked thought
- A blocked action
- Impaired perceptual ability
- Bound energy
- Blocked joy

To cure ourselves of chronic muscular pain, or chronic emotional pain (however you look at it -- it's the same thing), we must identify all your mind body pain units, and become conscious of them. For each, we must identify its chronic muscular tension in your body, its emotion, the moment in your life that caused it, the thoughts behind it, and so on.

Looking at mind body pain units in this way is the process of "introspection". It is asking "What do I feel, and why do I feel it?"

We must analyse what is true, and what is not true. We must experience all the blocked emotions. We must go through the protective "fear layer" guarding those emotions. We must feel the physical pain in your muscles, in your heart, in your stomach, in your brain.

It's important at this point to address a number of issues, for which these Mind Body Pain Units are likely to be responsible (my opinion, thus far). We initiated our discussion with physical conditions - painful chronic muscular tensions. Though we could have just as easily initiated our discussion with mind-oriented conditions.

Anxiety, stress, psychosis, neurosis, depression, obsession, compulsion, mania, addiction, sadism, masochism. The list is exceptionally long. These are all simply accumulations of many or extremely powerful (or both) Mind Body Pain Units of a common type. Either anxious, psychotic, neurotic, depressive, obsessive, compulsive, manic, addictive, sadistic, masochistic or so on.

To suggest that these do not come from a person's experience and their physical, emotional and analytical response to experience is, frankly, absurd. Yes of course, the brain can be poisoned or physically damaged, but in all cases where a person has not ingested poisonous chemicals, or had their brain irreparably damaged by physical trauma, it's clear that these conditions are caused by painful moments in the person's life, forming Mind Body Pain Units.

**Summary of this chapter:**

- For any experience, we have the choice to become conscious of it, or to evade it
- Becoming conscious of experience is neither immediate, nor automatic
- Becoming conscious takes effort, time, intellectual strength and willingness to feel pain
- A lifetime of evasion results in overflowing Mind Body Pain Units

**Exercise 8: Legs in the Air, or "Baby Legs"**

Lay on your back and put your legs in the air. The only requirement of this exercise is that your feet and legs are up off the ground. Now you may explore a lot of the mobility of your hip joints.

You may bend your knees or keep them straight. You may move one leg differently to the other. Your hip joint is a ball and socket joint, so you have a lot of freedom to move.

If you stay doing this exercise for a prolonged period, you will most likely experience a lot of burning tension in your hip flexors and lower abs. Also pay attention to your lower back. If your lower back is hurting, you should probably do something to make the exercise easier.

Be aware that you're not "strengthening" the musculature. That may be a secondary, possibly unavoidable, outcome, but it is not the intention. The intention is to get to know the muscles of your hips, and your core.

Learn the nature of the chronic muscular tensions that make this exercise more difficult than it should be and learn to optimize your movement patterns to make the movement more efficient, comfortable and joyful.

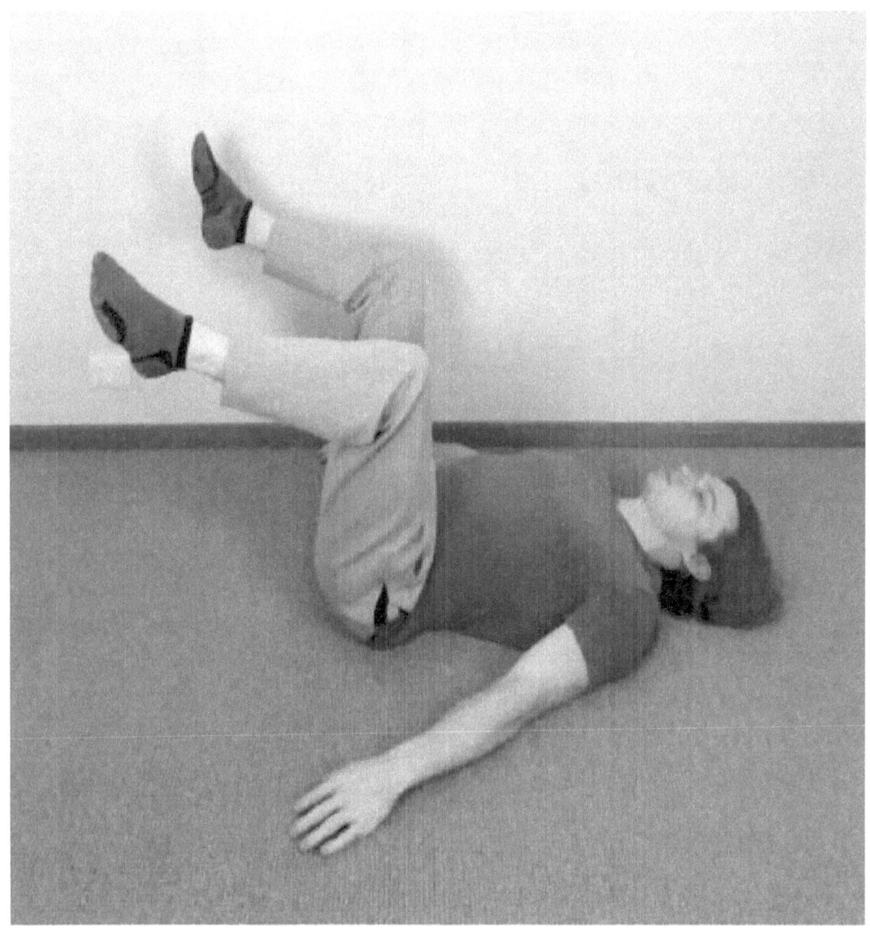

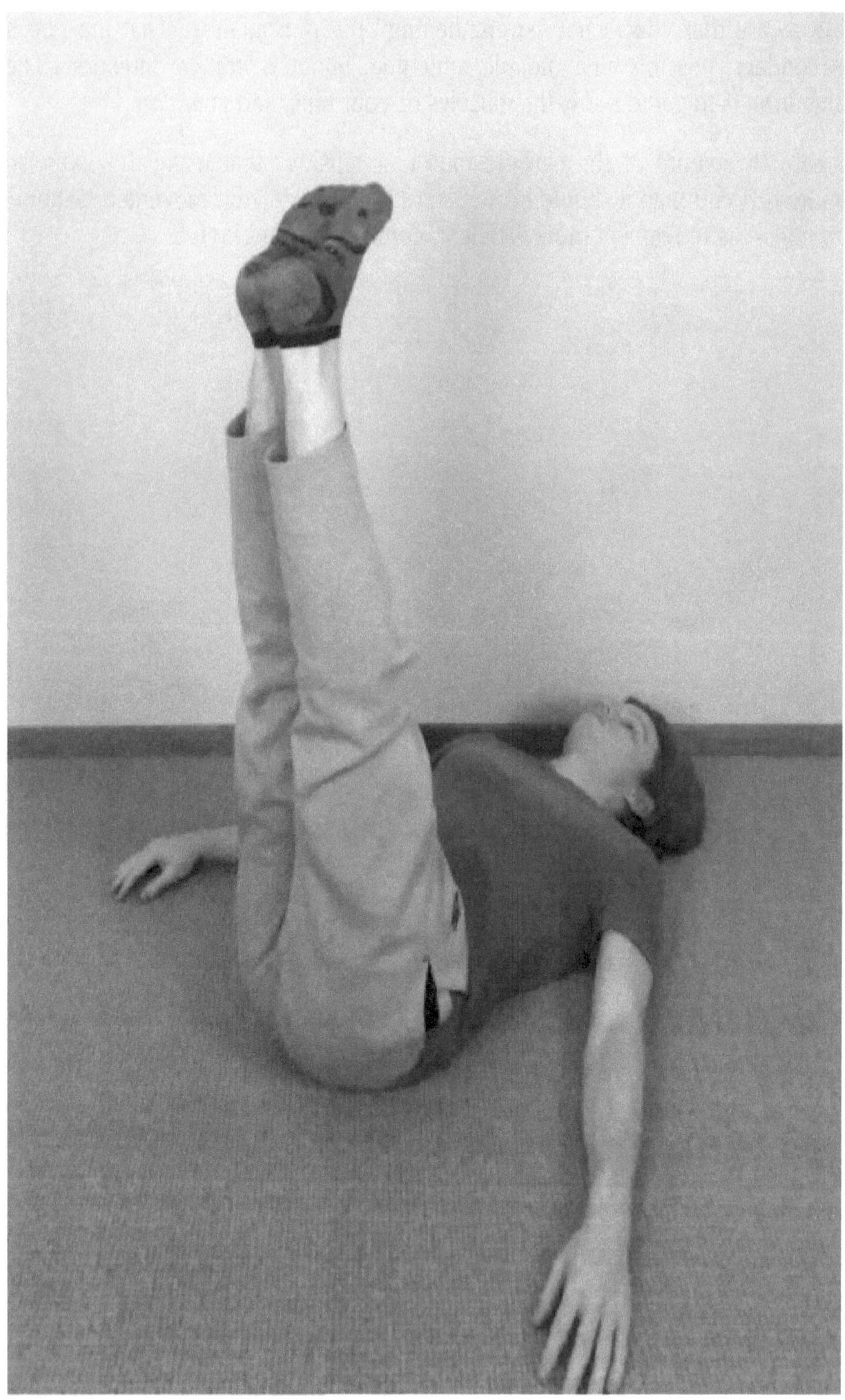

# CHAPTER 9: INTRODUCING "CONSCIOUS MOVEMENT"

As soon as you resolve any unique Mind-Body Pain Unit, its physical pain will be permanently gone, as will the fear of that physical pain, because it no longer exists. Full use and control of the previously affected musculature will immediately return. Joy will flow more readily through the body.

The energy that was being wasted on tensing your muscles will no longer be bound to that chore and become available to you. Your mind will become clearer and more rational and you will become more present and conscious. That moment will no longer control your actions or prevent you from doing what you want to do. You will have more power to live your life how you wish.

And when you do this for every single Mind-Body Pain Unit, you will simultaneously restore your complete potential. Potential for feeling, for moving, for perceiving, for thinking, for achieving, for living. You will wield the full power of your mind and your body and be able to do things that once seemed impossible.

The ultimate question is -- what's the best way to resolve Mind-Body Pain Units? Most methods proposed thus far are bad because they target either the body, or the mind, but almost never both.

Stretching, massage, physiotherapy, calisthenics, gymnastics, yoga, martial arts, weights, exercise -- these are all purely physical approaches that don't even begin to reference the mind. And they are always instructed by people who have no useful understanding of the mind. Someone who has many Mind-Body Pain Units, may seemingly improve their body function by doing these, though they'll do it by finding ways to evade their existing pain, and thus build even more protective layers around their pain.

Without the mind and emotions involved, any "progress" is illusory.

Psychology, psychotherapy, Buddhism, meditation, Dianetics, self-development, Objectivism. These are far better than the physical approaches. While they can get people good results, even great results, people often "plateau", and some people make no progress at all, because they lack the physical component to work with the experience of fear and painful emotion, and the release and reactivation of musculature.

There are some mind-body methodologies out there, including Bioenergetics, Beyond Systems, Developmental Movement, Qigong, though having explored them in complete depth, I have found them to be either incomplete, or too complex to understand, and ultimately not a person's best path toward complete resolution of Mind Body Pain Units.

Having studied every single field mentioned in great detail, some 20,000 hours or more, to resolve my own pain, I will now present to you a synthesis, taking the best parts from each. You may try this method at your own leisure, and I think it will offer you the best chance available at resolving your own situation.

The activity that eventually yields these outcomes is called "Conscious Movement".

Conscious Movement is a crucial daily activity for any person who wishes to move beyond muscular pain or emotional pain (which are really the same thing), or any person who wishes to "become more conscious".

If you could begin spending just 15 minutes a day doing one new activity to radically improve your life, it would be Conscious Movement.

Let me paint a complete picture for you by looking at the activity through a dozen or so lenses:

Conscious movement is contracting and relaxing your muscles. It's opening, closing and rotating your joints. It's moving your whole body. While being conscious of your body, your emotions and your thoughts. Conscious Movement is exploring your muscles, your joints, your mobility, the tensions in your body, asking "What do I feel?", "Why do I feel it?"

Conscious Movement is lowering your defenses and allowing your movements to stimulate tensions in your muscles, which trigger emotions, thoughts, and memories from your past. Conscious movement is breaking apart old, habitual inefficient movement patterns and replacing them with comfortable, efficient, precise, low-tension movement patterns.

Conscious movement is explorative, investigative, meditative, introspective, contemplative. Conscious Movement invites painful emotions and painful thoughts to come into the light of your consciousness and reveal their secrets. Conscious Movement intentionally facilitates the complete processing of painful emotions and thoughts, and the instantaneous release of chronic muscular tension.

Conscious Movement isn't only the "best" solution to chronic muscular/emotional pain, it is the only solution, because it is, by definition, the act of working with your muscles, your emotions and your mind in one connected experience.

Whenever you're using a combined physical, emotional and mental approach, you are doing Conscious Movement, by definition. You are triggering the process of "consciousness".

All that lies between you and the release of all chronic pain from your life, is learning how to effectively do Conscious Movement. On the other side of that is physical comfort and wellbeing, and as I said in the beginning, a perfectly healthy emotional system, a mind without worry, stress or anxiety, a mind free from undeserved fear, guilt and regret, a clear mind, inhabiting a joyful body, living happily, and more energy than you've had in years.

After you have sufficient experience training your Conscious Movement abilities, you will be able to do the following ritual:

1) Do movements that stimulate the chronically tense musculature

2) Focus progressively deeper on any tensions that you perceive

3) Ask yourself "What do I feel?" and "Why do I feel it?"

4) Listen to the thoughts rumbling around in your subconscious

5) Explore and develop those thoughts

6) Return to memories of moments in which you first had these thoughts

7) Notice the emotions that these thoughts trigger

8) Continue stimulating the muscles

9) Allow the emotions to increase, no matter how scary or uncomfortable

10) Come to a full understanding of the physical pain, the memory, the emotion and the thoughts

11) Experience release of that conflict, with release of muscular and emotional pain

12) Move on to another tension

While this ritual describes the experience of a "release", this is only an outcome. I expect that very few people would be able to read this, and then immediately be able to perform it.

I trained under the instruction of Eero Westerberg approximately 6 months before I learned to perceive and control my muscles well enough to focus deeply on them and release a tension for the first time.

You may be able to do it already, though most people will need to train their conscious control and perception of their musculature before they are capable.

That's why the next chapter will provide instruction on how to reach a point where you can release tension/pain on command. Eventually you will be able to do that while simply resting in a comfortable lounge chair.

**Summary of this chapter:**

- Human faculties return as you resolve mind body pain units
- Conscious Movement does not "resolve pain", it is the process of resolving pain

- You can learn to release pain on command and totally free yourself
- Significant training may be required to learn to release pain (it's worth it)

## Exercise 9: Ballet 2nd Position in Front of a Wall

Stand in front of a wall with your legs turned outward approximately 45 degrees, and your toes touching the wall. The distance between your heels should, for the sake of simplicity, be approximately 10 inches, though it wouldn't really matter if you chose 2 inches, or 20 inches.

Place the palms of your hands on the wall somewhere above your head. Hold this position for an extended period of time. You can and should move your arms anywhere you like, as long as your palms remain touching the wall.

Turn your focus inward toward your alignment. This is an alignment exercise. Focus especially on your feet, your knees, your pelvis and your lower back. Try to find uncomfortable tensions in your position. Find where you are "holding" you are unnecessarily holding your muscles too tensely. Modify the pose to be more comfortable.

Ask yourself, "What is the extent of the gap between my alignment right now, and what my alignment could be in the future if I keep working at it?" … "What is alignment anyway, and how should I use my analytical mind to guide me toward it?"

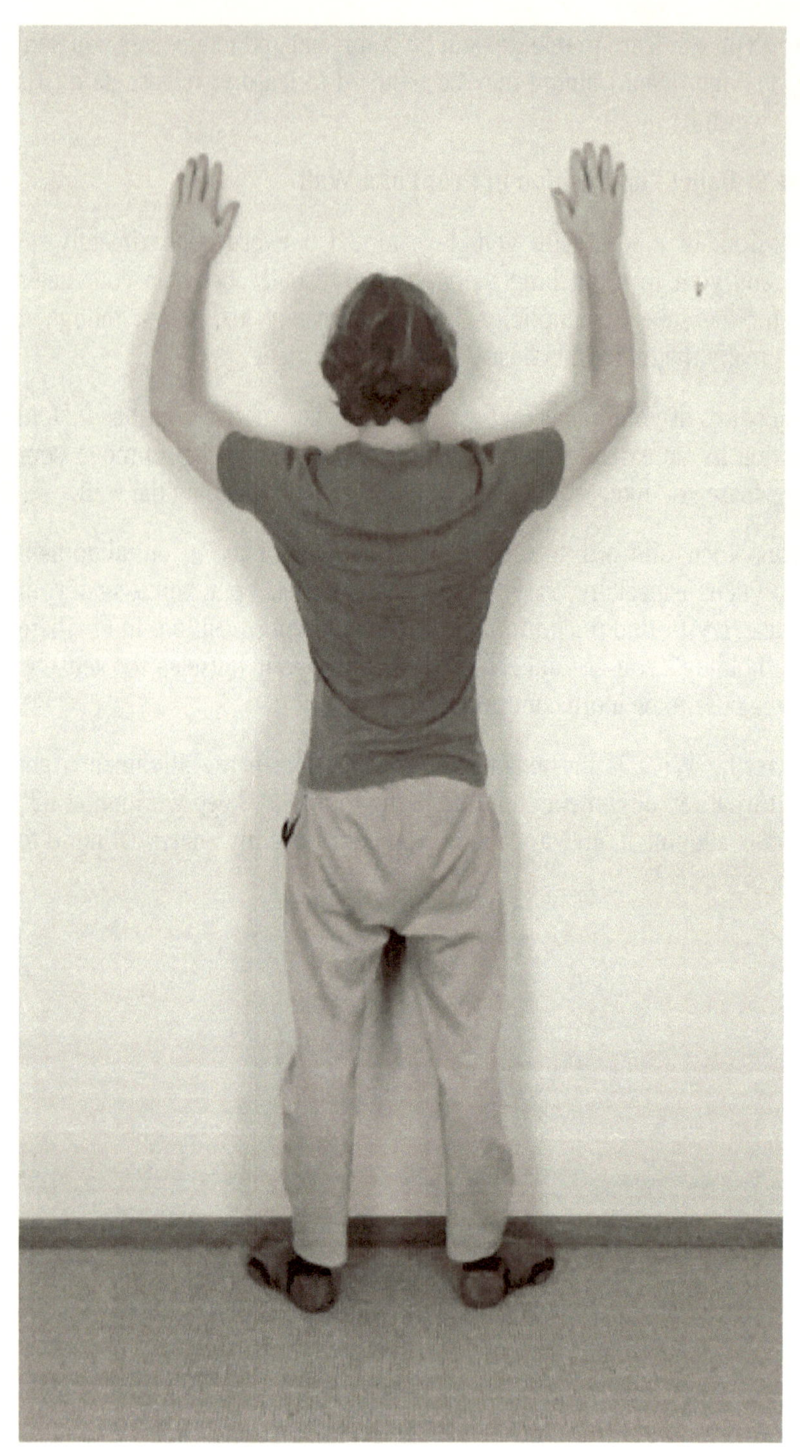

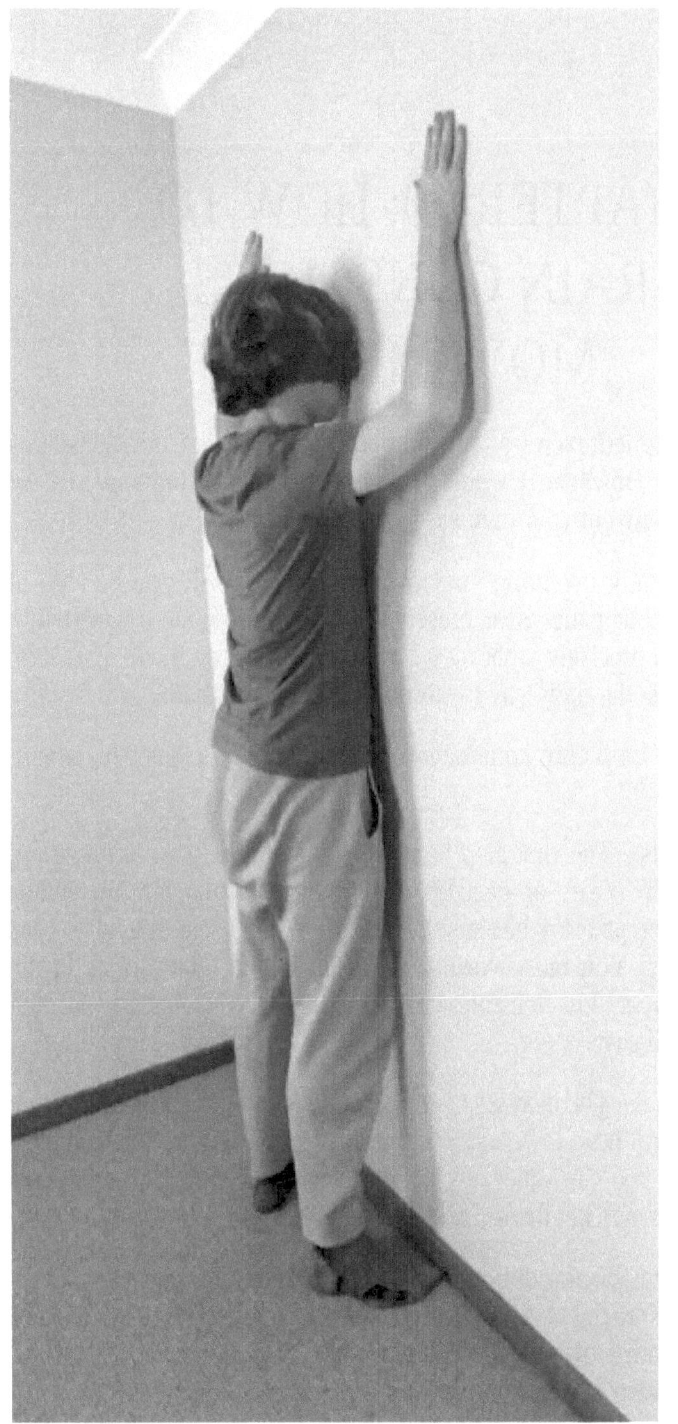

# CHAPTER 10: HOW TO TRAIN CONSCIOUS MOVEMENT

I have already supplied exercises in this book, which are of the Conscious Movement variety. However, I would like to conceptualize the approach so that you are able to invent your own exercises/movements.

Only by independently inventing your own movements will you be able to succeed, because your patterns of muscular tension are unique to your life. No one else knows precisely what they are, so only you can move, perceive, feel and think in just the right way to stimulate and release them.

I consider there to be 6 core components of training Conscious Movement, which are as follows:

1) Joint Movements - The first step is to learn the correct way to move the joints of your body. Years or decades of chronic muscular tension and/or incorrect movement patterns has resulted in your joints moving in a very "high tension" way. You must learn to open, close and rotate joints in the most energy efficient, low tension way so that your movements become noticeably light and easy.

2) Muscles Squeezes - The next step is to get in touch with muscle fibers that you probably haven't used in years. You must learn to use your mind-muscle connection so that you can squeeze your muscles, from the right angles and with the right focus, and get them working again.

These first two steps do not directly treat chronic muscular tension, though they are absolutely crucial as a foundation. They will give you the necessary awareness and control of your body to be able to perform the following techniques that actively remove chronic muscular tension.

3) The "Tension On, Tension Off" Technique - This is the technique I described earlier, in which you focus on a muscle, contracting it and relaxing it, while you open your mind to memories, emotions and thoughts, and resolve inner conflicts that come up.

4) Static Holds - Sometimes chronic muscular tensions are in deep muscles fibers that have become completely dormant, and you have lost the connection between your mind and those muscles entirely. The Static Hold technique is a simple matter of holding your body in a position for a length of time that tires out incorrect, inefficient patterns of muscular contraction, and forces dormant muscles to wake up and be on your team.

5) Free Form Conscious Movement - After you get the hang of Tension On, Tension Off, and Static Holds, you may begin to feel proficient at releasing chronic muscular tension, and you will be able to begin using an advanced method that will release tensions that you don't currently even know exist. In Free Form Conscious Movement, you begin in any position you like, and allow yourself to be guided, moment by moment, by your instincts.

You allow your entire mind to sync up with the muscular tension and your emotions, and allow your body complete freedom to move, as you explore your muscles, emotions and mind in a completely uninhibited way.

6) Integration into Life - The final step is to fully integrate what you learn into your life. That is, your moment to moment experience. You should learn mindsets to use your muscles, joints, emotions and mind in an optimum way in your everyday life, so that you feel great all the time, with enthusiasm and a bright outlook on life.

When all of these are sufficiently practiced, you will be able to sit in a comfortable chair, or lay down on a soft floor, and release painful tension on command.

It may take you years, perhaps even a decade to do it all, but it can happen. And as far as I know, Conscious Movement is by definition, the only path, because it is the only activity that involves the physical, the emotional and the mental, with the specific intention of releasing pain and becoming conscious.

**Summary of this Chapter:**

- There are 6 core components of training Conscious Movement
- Joint movements, muscles squeezes and static holds will build your perception
- Tension on, tension off will actively resolve pain
- Free form conscious movement, and integration into life will eventually come

**Exercise 10: Your Exercise**

One of the major themes of this book is "independence". The virtue of thinking for yourself and choosing your own actions.

The totality of your pain cannot be released by exercises that I invented for myself. I tried to give you exercises that are quite general, though ultimately you will need to create your own exercises, because your pain is specific to you.

So, for your 10th exercise, create your own. Try to notice what you alone think you should notice. Do whatever you think is rational.